11-99

CARING FOR HEALTH
History and Diversity

prepared by the U205 Course Team

 THE OPEN UNIVERSITY
Health and Disease   U205   Book VII
A Second Level Course

THE OPEN UNIVERSITY PRESS

The U205 Course Team

U205 is a course whose writing and production has been the joint effort of many hands: a 'core course team', colleagues who have written on specific aspects of the course but have not been involved throughout, editors, designers, and the BBC team.

Core course team

The following people have written or commented extensively on the whole course, been involved in all phases of its production and accept collective responsibility for its overall academic and teaching content.

Steven Rose (neurobiologist; course team chair; academic editor; Book VI coordinator)

Nick Black (community physician; Book IV coordinator; Book VIII coordinator)

Basiro Davey (immunologist; course manager; Book V coordinator)

Alastair Gray (health economist; Book III coordinator; Book VII coordinator)

Kevin McConway (statistician; Book I coordinator)

Jennie Popay (social policy analyst)

Phil Strong (medical sociologist; academic editor; Book II coordinator)

Other authors

The following authors have contributed to the overall development of the course and have taken responsibility for writing specific sections of it.

Lynda Birke (ethologist; author, Book V)

Eric Bowers (parasitologist; staff tutor)

David Boswell (sociologist; author, Book II)

Eva Chapman (psychotherapist; author, Book V)

Andrew Learmonth (geographer; course team chair 1983; author, Book III)

Rosemary Lennard (medical practitioner; author, Books IV and V)

Jim Moore (historian of science; author, Book II)

Sean Murphy (neurobiologist; author, Book VI)

Rob Ransom (developmental biologist; author, Book IV)

George Watts (historian; author, Book II)

The following people have assisted with particular aspects or parts of the course.

Steve Best (illustrator)

Sheila Constantinou (BBC production assistant)

Gerald Copp (editor)

Ann Hall (indexer)

Debbie Crouch (designer)

Mark Kesby (illustrator)

Liz Lane (editor)

Vic Lockwood (BBC producer)

Laurie Melton (librarian)

Peggy Stevens (course secretary)

Jacqueline Stewart (managing editor until January 1985)

Sue Walker (editor)

Peter Wright (editor)

External Consultant

Robert Dingwall (sociologist) Centre for Socio-legal Studies, Wolfson College, Oxford.

External assessors

Course assessor

Alwyn Smith, President, Faculty of Community Medicine of the Royal Colleges of Physicians; Professor of Epidemiology and Social Oncology, University of Manchester.

Book VII Assessors

Brian Abel-Smith, Professor of Social Administration, London School of Economics and Political Science.

Gordon Horobin, MRC Medical Sociology Unit, Aberdeen.

Peter West, Health Economics Research Unit, University of Aberdeen.

The Open University Press, Walton Hall, Milton Keynes MK7 6AA.

First published 1985. Reprinted 1988, 1991. Copyright © 1985 The Open University.

Designed by the Graphic Design Group of the Open University.

Printed and bound in Great Britain by Mackays of Chatham PLC, Chatham, Kent

ISBN 0 335 15056 X

This book forms part of an Open University course. The complete list of books in the course is printed on the back cover.

For general availability of supporting material referred to in this book please write to: Open University Educational Enterprises Limited, 12 Cofferidge Close, Stony Stratford, Milton Keynes, MK11 1BY, Great Britain.

Further information on Open University courses may be obtained from The Admissions Office, The Open University, P.O. Box 48, Walton Hall, Milton Keynes, MK7 6AB.

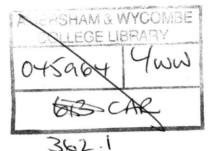

About this book

A note for the general reader

Caring for Health: History and Diversity is the seventh of a series of books on the subject of health and disease. The book is designed so that it can be read on its own, like any other textbook, or studied as part of U205 *Health and Disease*, a second level course for Open University students. As well as the eight textbooks and a Course Reader, *Health and Disease: A Reader,** the course consists of eleven TV programmes and five audiocassettes plus various supplementary materials.

Open University students will receive an *Introduction and Guide* to the course, which sets out a study plan for the year's work. This is supplemented where appropriate in the text by more detailed directions for OU students; these study comments at the beginning of chapters are boxed for ease of reference. Also, in the text you will find instructions to refer to the Course Reader. It is quite possible to follow the argument without reading the articles referred to, although your understanding will be enriched if you do so. Major learning objectives are listed at the end of each chapter along with questions that allow students to assess how well they are achieving those objectives. The index includes key words (in bold type) which can be looked up easily as an aid to revision as the course proceeds. There is also a further reading list for those who wish to pursue certain aspects of study beyond the limits of this book.

A guide for OU students

In *Caring for Health: History and Diversity* we introduce the subject of health care. The book has two main themes: first, that the phrase 'health care' in practice embraces an extraordinarily wide range of activities, and second, that these can best be understood by adopting a comparative and historical perspective.

The book falls roughly into two main parts preceded by an introduction. Chapters 2–5 set out a broad historical picture of the development of health care, and Chapters 6–9 explore the diversity of health care in the present world.

The time allowed for studying Book VII is four weeks or 40 hours. The table overleaf gives a more detailed breakdown to help you pace your studies. You need not follow it slavishly but do not allow yourself to fall behind. If you find a section of the work difficult, do what you can at this stage, and then rework the material at the end of your study of this book.

*Black, Nick *et al.* (eds) (1984) *Health and Disease: A Reader*, Open University Press.

Study time for Book VII (total 40 hours)

Chapter	Time/hours	Course Reader	Time/hours	TV/Audio Tapes	Time/hours	Total per week/hours
1	1					
2	5					} 10½
3	4½					
4	7½					} 10½
5	3					
6	2½	Bowling and Cartwright (1982)	¾			
7	2½				1½	} 10¾
8	3½	Ramesh and Hyma (1981)	¾	TV and		
9	2½	Werner (1978)	¾	related audio		} 8¼
10	1¼					

Assessment   There is a TMA (tutor-marked assignment) associated with this book; three hours have been allowed for its completion.

Acknowledgements
The Course Team wishes to thank the following for their advice and contributions:

Sheila Adam (community physician) North-West Thames Regional Health Authority.

John Ashton (community physician) Department of Community Health, University of Liverpool.

Mel Bartley (sociologist) Department of Social Administration, University of Edinburgh.

Graham Burchell (philosopher) Westminster College of Education, Oxford.

Hilary Graham (sociologist) Department of Applied Social Studies, University of Bradford.

Dave Gee (National Health and Safety Officer) General, Municipal, Boilermakers and Associated Trades Union.

Barbara Harrison (medical sociologist) Department of Social Sciences, Polytechnic of the South Bank.

Irvine Loudon (general practitioner/historian) Wellcome Unit for the History of Medicine, University of Oxford.

Anne Murcott (sociologist) Department of Sociology, University of Cardiff; Department of Psychological Medicine, Welsh National School of Medicine.

Tom Patterson (historian) Wellcome Unit for the History of Medicine, University of Oxford.

Margaret Pelling (historian) Wellcome Unit for the History of Medicine, University of Oxford.

Emilie Savage-Smith (historian) Gustave E. von Grunebaum Center for Near Eastern Studies, University of California, Los Angeles.

Charles Webster (historian) Wellcome Unit for the History of Medicine, University of Oxford.

Paul Weindling (historian) Wellcome Unit for the History of Medicine, University of Oxford.

Contents

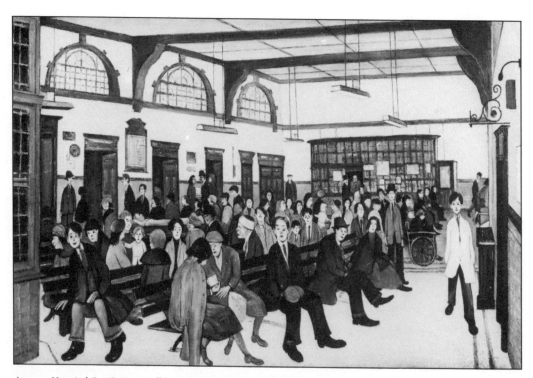

Ancoats Hospital Out-Patient Hall by L. S. Lowry (1952). Situated in north-west Manchester, the Ancoats Hospital was built in the 1870s with money raised by voluntary donations and bequests. Nationalised in 1948, it continued as a general hospital in the NHS until 1982, when it was converted for use as a specialised orthopaedic unit.

1

Caring for health: an introduction

This book is about health care, as it exists in the modern world, and as it has been in the past. But what do we mean by health care? In modern language and thought, health care has become a phrase attached to a specialised set of activities, provided by people who are highly trained for people who are sick, and concentrated in a health care 'sector' of society — a health service, a health care system, or a health care industry.

The 'health care sector' is very visible in industrialised countries: its vehicles rush through the streets with flashing lights and wailing sirens; its workers (particularly doctors and nurses) wear distinctive clothes and feature constantly in TV serials, newspapers, and films; its buildings include some of the most complex and expensive erected in the twentieth century. We all come into contact with this health care sector, often at critical times in our lives: birth, accident, illness and death, and so it involves many of our profoundest hopes and fears. Around one in twenty of us earns a living by providing it. And finally, it lays claim to national resources on an immense scale in the world's wealthiest countries. In the USA, for example, 300 000 million dollars were spent on health care in 1982, an almost unimaginable sum, and larger in fact than the entire national income of China, which contains one fifth of the Earth's population.

There are lots of reasons, therefore, why anyone interested in health care should focus on the health care sector. In this book, however, we begin by throwing overboard the idea that health care is defined by this health care sector. Why should we do this? Broadly, there are three reasons.

1 The great bulk of the attention to health and ill-health that we give and receive is *outside* the health care sector.

2 The health care sector embodies one particular view of health and disease, and one particular kind of response. It is in fact the *personal* health care sector, organised around the bringing together of medical staff and individual patient; it is, in a sense, a personal tinkering trade. But there are other conceptions of health care.

3 Health care is part of society, and is subject to an enormous variety of influences. Therefore, it can only be understood in its social context: viewed in isolation, it is not an intelligible field of study.

Consider first the argument that the main source of health care lies outside the health care sector. Table 1.1 shows the results of a survey of diseases and disorders among the population of part of London in 1967.

☐ What does this table reveal?

■ In all the categories of ill-health listed, the majority of sufferers (two in three on average) did not seek the attention of the health care sector.

Table 1.1 Ill-health in Bermondsey and Southwark, 1967

Disease category	Proportion of population suffering from disease in this category (%)	Proportion of sufferers who had never taken these complaints to the doctor (%)
Respiratory system	26	63
Mental, psychoneurotic and personality	21	80
Bones and organs of movement	15	61
Digestive system	11	78
Nervous system and sense organs	8	59
Skin and cellular tissue	5	73
Circulatory system	4	58
Accidents	3	78

(Source: Wadsworth, Butterfield and Blaney, 1968)

Most health care is unpaid and usually provided in the home. This is as true of the present as it was of the past, and will almost certainly continue to be true of the future. We will be referring to this form of health care as *lay health care*, and to doctors, hospitals, nurses and so on as *formal health care*. In practice, however, there is seldom a hard and fast distinction, as this story illustrates:

> I was twelve years of age ... the operation was done on the kitchen table. The nurse came and the doctor and I've so much of my rib taken, it's cut down here and down my back and it was done on the kitchen table. The nurse came and attended to the wound for several weeks. They gave me an anaesthetic. All had to take place during the housework and the elder ones coming in for their meals ... The doctor said, 'Mrs T, this is ideal for the job, you couldn't have a better table'. There was no talk of going into hospital. There was no walls scrubbed, but everything had to be clean and I remember mother saying that the nurse said, 'Well you've got everything just right'. They had a bucket for the blood. (Cited in Roberts, 1980, p.38)

☐ Which term — 'lay' or 'formal' — do you think best describes the care that the girl in this quote received in a Lancashire house in 1912?
■ You probably had some difficulty in deciding, as there were elements of both types of care. The operation certainly took place in a lay setting — a scrubbed kitchen table amidst housework and cooking. However, the people involved included both laity (her mother) and formal carers (a doctor and a nurse).

Most formal care in industrialised countries now occurs in a formal setting such as hospitals, clinics, or health centres, which are easily identifiable by their architecture, furnishings, and even their smell. But doctors and nurses visit patients in their own homes; ambulance staff often tend people out of doors; and faith healers may hold meetings in public halls. The location of lay care is equally diverse. In addition to the domestic setting, it takes place in formal institutions such as hospitals. For example, in the UK it is common practice for parents to help care for their children in hospital, while throughout the Third World such involvement is a feature of virtually all types of hospital care. The setting is therefore of little value in distinguishing lay from formal care.

Both lay and formal care are concerned with three main areas of activity: the maintenance of health and prevention of disease; the diagnosis and treatment of illness; and the support and care of those who are chronically ill, infirm or disabled. These activities illustrate the *interdependence* of lay and formal care, but again they provide little to distinguish the two.

Formal care can probably be identified most easily by

the people who provide it: these people are generally recognised by the community as 'healers' having specialised knowledge or skills; and they are *paid*, in cash or in kind, for the services that they perform. They need not necessarily therefore be legally qualified or registered. Throughout the history of human societies, formal carers have emerged: witches, wise women, shamans, bone-setters, yogin, barber-surgeons, nurses, pharmacists, doctors ... the list is almost endless.

In contrast, lay providers — including relatives, friends and neighbours whose advice and help may at times be sought — are not generally recognised as possessing special skills nor would they receive payment for their efforts.

There is an important point to be made about the people providing lay health care. You may have noticed in the story from Lancashire quoted above that it was 'Mrs T' that the nurse complimented for getting 'everything just right'. It is very unlikely that Mr T would have been involved in the preparations, for to a very large extent lay health care was and still is women's work. But women are also represented in large numbers within the formal sector, disproportionately in lower status occupations. So although the gender of the health carers is not a way of distinguishing between lay and formal care, it is an important theme of all health care, and will recur throughout this book.

When we look at health care, therefore, the main point is that it is essential to include not just the formal health care sector, but also lay care, for the two are inextricably connected, and each continually influences the other.

The second reason for widening the horizons of this book beyond the health care sector is that the *personal* health care provided by this sector is only one particular form of health care. In fact, health care has been envisaged in a quite different way, as:

> the science and art of preventing disease, prolonging life, and promoting physical health and efficiency through organized community efforts for the sanitation of the environment, the control of community infections ... and the development of the social machinery which will ensure to every individual in the community a standard of living adequate for the maintenance of health. (Winslow, 1920, p.30)

☐ How does this view differ from that of personal health care?
■ With personal health care, the patient is an individual, and intervention is at a personal level; according to the view quoted above, the 'patient' is the community or population as a whole, and intervention occurs at a social level.

A powerful alternative to personal health care, therefore, is the notion of *public health*. Indeed, most Europeans daily

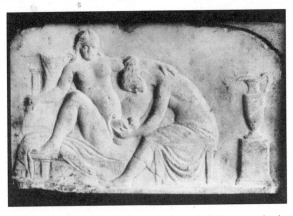

Figure 1.1 Midwifery. (a) A Roman bas-relief showing a birth-scene with a midwife in attendance. In Greece, Rome, and indeed throughout most of recorded history, midwifery has generally been undertaken by women. Two midwives — Shiprah and Puah — are discussed in the Book of Exodus.

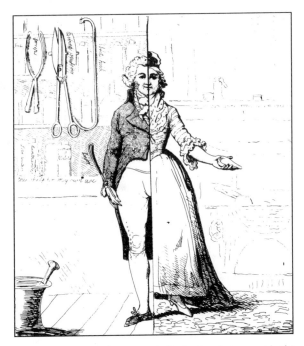

(b) By 1625 a new word was in use in England — the 'man-midwife' — and such work seemed for a time likely to become a largely male preserve (in the USA it did). The cartoon is from a book published in 1793 by S. W. Forbes entitled *Man-Midwifery Dissected*. Behind the male half-figure are bottles of 'love-water' and other potions allegedly used on patients as sexual stimulants.

pay tribute to the achievements of public health when they run the tap, use the toilet, eat a meal, or simply breathe the air. Equally, many millions of Africans, Asians and Latin Americans daily pay a heavy toll of sickness and death for the absence of public health.

According to the definition quoted above, public health encompasses many things that are far removed from the formal health care sector: sewage, sanitation, industrial safety legislation, income maintenance, etc. A sizeable place has also been made for discussing such things in this book, for it is probable that public health care if anything has been more important than personal health care in influencing disease and ill-health.

The third reason for not confining the scope of the book to the health care sector alone is that health care is subject to a variety of wider influences. Three in particular stand out: (a) the burden of disease and its changing pattern; (b) shifts in medical knowledge and in views of disease; and (c) social, political and economic forces.* In this book we are going to concentrate on the third, the social, political and economic factors that have influenced the way health care has developed. (You should, however, bear in mind the other two, and at times we shall refer to examples of how changes in both the pattern of disease and medical knowledge have exerted vitally important influences on health care.)

What are those social, political and economic influences? Changes of government, whether by election, revolution, or military coup, often signal abrupt changes in the direction and form of health services. In a letter to his brother shortly before becoming Chancellor of the Exchequer, Lloyd George noted that 'it is time we did something that appealed straight to the people . . . it will, I think, help to stop the electoral rot . . .' That 'something' took the form of the introduction of old age pensions in 1908 and of National Health Insurance in 1911. Changes in technology also create health care changes: items that are now commonplace and taken for granted like the telephone and motor car completely transformed American medical practice in the space of a few years. Newer technologies, such as computers, are having effects at the moment. Religious attitudes and beliefs affect health care in numerous ways, from attitudes to death and disease to the provision of hospitals and the recruitment of nurses. Medical students still travel from one country to another (until the 1970s, for example, from Denmark to England) to study anatomy, because dissection is banned on religious grounds in their own country. The size of the health care sector appears to be much more closely related to economic wealth than to the amount of ill-health. The structure of the

* (a) is discussed in detail in The Open University (1985) *The Health of Nations*, The Open University Press (U205 *Health and Disease*, Book III); (b) is discussed in detail in The Open University (1985) *Medical Knowledge: Doubt and Certainty*, The Open University Press (U205 *Health and Disease*, Book II).

family has some bearing on the need for institutions such as hospitals and homes, as well as influencing the provision of lay care, and so on. The list could be extended, but the essential point is that health care does not exist in a vacuum and cannot be studied as if it did.

So this book is about the health care sector, but not only about that. The broader subject of the book is caring for health, the many different forms this takes, and the way caring for health fits into human society.

History and diversity

Caring for health comprises a variety of different activities in any society, but these activities also vary a lot between one society and another, and between one period of history and another. Take, for example, hospitals. Writing in the sixteenth century, the English poet Edmund Spenser used the word in the following way:

> They spy'd a goodly castle, plac'd
> Foreby a river in a pleasant dale,
> Which chusing for that evening's hospital,
> They thither marched.
> (*The Faerie Queene*)

☐ What sense is conveyed of the hospital in this passage?

■ The word is used to denote a place of shelter, refuge or hospitality.

It could be argued that, although hospitals are no longer used by travellers for overnight stops, some are still used extensively to provide refuge for people who are not temporarily sick, but are simply old, or homeless, or handicapped and have nowhere else to go to be looked after. Nevertheless, the meaning of the word 'hospital' has changed and now denotes a place exclusively for the use of sick people. And it is not just the meaning of the word that varies between time and place: the nurses inside hospitals, characteristically women in modern Europe, were for long almost exclusively men in many Middle Eastern and African countries, as were the patients. The number of people working in hospitals can also vary widely, even between quite similar countries: Scotland, for example, has 50 per cent more hospital doctors per head of population than England.

This diversity, encountered in all aspects of health care, is often ignored in the desire to simplify things, and normally caring for health is examined in only one society at one point in time. The well-worn cliché about insular attitudes in Victorian Britain, 'Storms in the channel — the Continent Isolated', did not vanish with the Victorians and is found not only in Britain. Home and abroad, familiar and foreign, domestic and strange, all too frequently lead to another division: relevant and irrelevant. This book takes

the opposite view: that it is important to look closely at different ways of caring for health in the present and the past. History and diversity are therefore the two constant themes of the book. There are a number of reasons for taking this view. Let's take history first.

Health care is full of instances where history is used (or abused) to support particular points of view. The medical profession has created the notion of the Hippocratic Oath, alluding to a tradition of medical ethics stretching back to ancient Greece that in fact never existed in that form. Contemporary debates in health care on 'medicalisation', on 'natural' medicine, on 'institutionalisation' or on the 'cost crisis' all draw implicitly on a version of history where the past was somehow quite different — whether better or worse — than the present.

Yet we know that there was concern in nineteenth-century hospitals about the rapidly escalating cost of leeches, that auditors were compulsorily placed in London's medieval hospitals to try to curb scandalous extravagances, that in 1657 the militia in Paris were ordered to hunt down beggars and confine them to city institutions. Four years later around 5 000–6 000 people had been thus 'institutionalised'. What we make of these facts is a different matter — they do not prove or disprove very much when taken in isolation. But the essential point is that most debates in contemporary health care draw on the past, sometimes acknowledging that they do, but often not.

The fact that contemporary debates often draw on versions of the past is only one reason for looking at history, however. Above all there is the fact that contemporary health care is the *consequence* of its past: the buildings, the ideas, the techniques, the occupations and the institutions. The structure and objectives of the National Health Service in the UK, for example, were a response to the past as well as a plan for the future, and cannot really be understood except in relation to what went before.

Or consider the following two descriptions of a hospital and a public health infrastructure:

> the hospital had an outpatient department and five sections each for a different class of ailments. A surgical ward of ten beds was provided for patients with fractures and wounds, a second ward of eight beds was assigned to patients with acute infectious diseases ... twelve beds in another ward were reserved for women ... each ward had no less than two physicians, three assistants and several orderlies. The women's ward had a woman physician in addition. (Rosen, 1963, p.5)

> Mechanical constructions answering purposes which we should now call sanitary, had made considerable progress ... there was an elaborate system of

drainage, no doubt essentially rain water drainage, in the basement ... a square brick-built main channel which ran, at three feet depth beneath the pavement ... to discharge itself into the river ... and opening into that channel, a contributary pipe-drain of baked clay from almost every chamber of the place. (Simon, 1890, p.10)

☐   When, do you think, the hospital and the sanitary works described may date from?

■   The hospital was Byzantine, opened in 1136 in Constantinople (Istanbul), and the sanitation system was constructed in Nineveh (in modern-day Iraq) over 3 000 years ago.

Again, it is difficult to understand the present unless we know something about how the present is different from the past, and that means taking a historical view. History, then, is not something that is redundant and dead, but rather is a dimension of the present which contains an enormous amount of data, experience, and collective wisdom.

The same reasons exist for examining the diversity of health care in the contemporary world. Specific comparisons are always being made by people for particular reasons: for example, to make claims that a country is spending too much or too little on health care, or that a country's standards of health care are better or worse than elsewhere. Lloyd George when British Prime Minister made comparisons between Britain and Germany to find ideas for reforming health care; the American Medical Association in the 1940s made comparisons with the British National Health Service to find ideas for avoiding reform in American health care. Selective comparison can be a powerful way of making propaganda, but if it is done more systematically it can be a powerful way of making sense of health care in the contemporary world, and a defence against the distortions which selective comparison inevitably entails.

Second, it is simply much easier to understand the nature of health care if comparisons are made between different societies. Comparisons, by revealing similarities and differences in the health care patterns of different societies, help to separate the common factors influencing health care from the factors unique to time and place.

Third, the sheer diversity of providing health care offers the opportunity to find better ways of doing things: from the way diseases are tackled to the way doctors are paid, lay carers are supported, or public health services provided.

In adopting a historical perspective, this book is not pretending to evaluate systematically a range of contemporary debates in light of the evidence from the past: that would be a mammoth task. The intention is to look more closely at the historical evidence that has to be taken into account before making any generalisations about health care in the present. That is the purpose of Chapters 2 to 5. And in adopting a comparative perspective, the book is not claiming to have found a catalogue of 'better ways of doing things'; the intention is simply to demonstrate that there is extraordinary diversity in health care, and this should be welcomed for the things that can be learned from it, and not avoided for the generalisations that awkward facts might impart. Chapters 6 to 9 of the book explore this diversity.

The concluding chapter returns to the themes of this introduction, using the material in the rest of the book to discuss in more detail the reasons why we cannot understand health care unless all forms of caring for health are recognised, and their history and diversity examined.

Finally, 'what is the use of a book', thought Alice, 'without pictures or conversations!' You will find only a few conversations in this book, but we have been able to include pictures. They are not solely illustrations of points made in the text, but often contain much information in their own right. They too have stories to tell.

2
Origins of European health care

This and the following three chapters examine the history of health care; they are intended to provide an account of the main developments in four *periods* of history, namely, (i) from the world of Greek and Roman antiquity to the end of the Middle Ages (Chapter 2), (ii) the early modern period from 1500 to 1800 (Chapter 3), (iii) the period from 1800 to the eve of the Second World War (Chapter 4), and (iv) from the Second World War to the present (Chapter 5). You are not expected to memorise a large number of actual dates or details, but rather to concentrate on the main developments. You may find it useful, therefore, to look at the objectives for each chapter before reading the text, and to keep these objectives in mind during your studies.

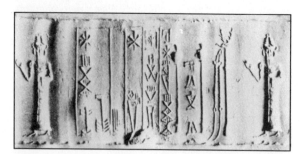

Figure 2.1 Sumerian clay documents were signed by rolling an engraved cylinder over them while wet. This one belonged to a physician from Lagash, and dates from around 3000 BC. The figure represents Iru, a form taken by the god of pestilence and disease, Nergal. It is now in the Louvre.

Before the Greeks and Romans, there were many major civilisations, to the south and east, which had already developed the medical art. The Sumerian is the world's oldest civilisation, which began in the Tigris and Euphrates valleys around 4000 BC, and had well-developed medical occupations (Figure 2.1). So too had the Egyptians, whose doctors were priests trained in temple medical schools. The world's oldest known surgical textbook is Egyptian and dates from around 1500 BC.

The history of European health care, however, is taken normally to have begun with the Greeks and in particular with the physician Hippocrates, who was born on the island of Cos near modern Turkey around 450 BC and who died 'at a great age' at Larissa in Thessaly* (these and other places referred to in this and the following chapter are shown in Figure 2.2). We start here because it is in Greece that the first essentially naturalistic approach to health and disease was developed in European medicine.

☐ What is meant by a 'naturalistic', as opposed to a 'supernatural', approach to health and disease?

■ A naturalistic approach holds that health and disease can be explained and understood in terms of natural events and forces, whereas a supernatural approach invokes divine or magical forces that are not of this world.†

Greece — the emergence of naturalism
To understand how naturalistic physicians arose as a powerful and influential group, we need first to consider wider aspects of the Greek civilisation. The key to Greek culture was the city-state or *polis*, from which English derives the terms 'political' and 'police'. By the eighth

---

*The lifetime dates of key people mentioned in the text are given in the index to this book.
†Naturalistic and supernatural approaches to health and disease are considered in much greater detail in *Medical Knowledge: Doubt and Certainty, ibid.*, Chapters 2 and 3 (U205 Book II).

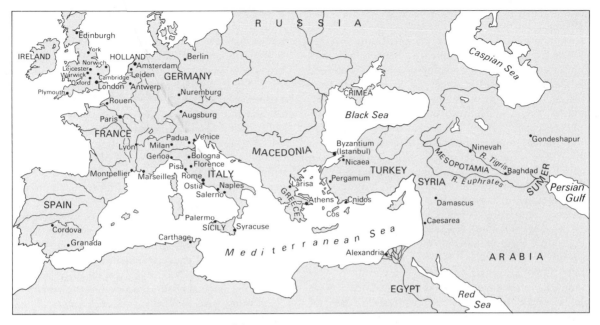

Figure 2.2 A map of Europe, the Mediterranean and the Near East.

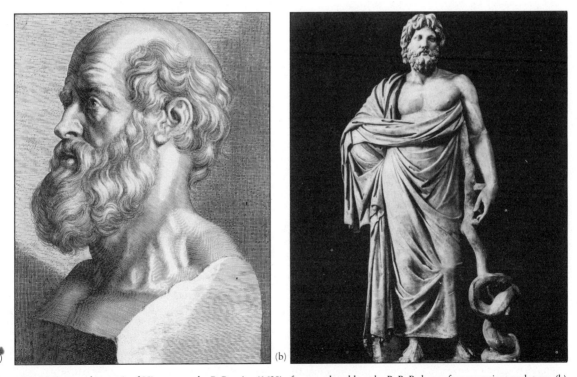

Figure 2.3 (a) Engraved portrait of Hippocrates by P. Pontius (1638) after a sculpted bust by P. P. Rubens after an ancient sculpture. (b) Statue of Aesculapius (Asklepios), the Greek god of healing, now in the Lateran Museum, Rome. The serpent (Coluber longissimus (Aesculapius)) has been the emblem of the art of healing from the Sumerian period to the present.

century BC a series of independent Greek cities had developed, and over the next two centuries they proceeded to colonise areas of southern Italy and Sicily, the Black Sea and the French Mediterranean coast, founding such cities as Marseilles, Naples (*nea-polis* or new city), Syracuse and Byzantium. A complex system of international trade developed between these far-flung states. The biggest cities, such as Athens, which eventually grew to a quarter of a million people, became increasingly rich and powerful. Then, in the fifth century BC, there occurred in addition to this economic transformation a scientific, intellectual and artistic revolution. Not just Hippocrates but Socrates, Plato, Democritus, Pericles, Aristophanes, Euripedes and Sophocles were all born in this century. It was at this time that we find the origins of modern medicine.

The medical profession was consciously forming itself into an organised group, and was trying to stake out a territory for itself while fending off others such as philosophers and priests. Greek medicine had no hospitals of any sort: there were temples in honour of Aesculapius, the healer god, and patients could go to shelter there for months or even years, but attention was focused on their faith rather than their bodies. The training of physicians was quite tightly tied to medical schools, the best-known being at Cos (the Coan school) and at nearby Cnidos (the Cnidian school). It was with the Coan school that Hippocrates was associated, but the body of writing now referred to as the *Hippocratic Corpus* was essentially the medical school library and not the work of one person.

Having become acquainted with the medical theories and body of knowledge on offer at medical school, the young physician would normally embark on a career by travelling with a master physician, whom he (they were all men) would serve as an apprentice.

☐ What reasons can you think of that might induce Greek physicians to have a travelling career?
■ In the first place, there were no institutions such as hospitals to offer posts. Second, there would be too few patients for too many physicians in the vicinity of the medical schools. And third, the many far-flung Greek city-states offered a potentially lucrative practice.

Part of the *Hippocratic Corpus* consists of seven books entitled *Epidemics*, and it has been suggested that the word '*epidemiai*' originally meant not outbreaks of infectious disease in a particular area, but rather the visit of a physician to an area, no doubt viewed as an attractive irony by present day therapeutic nihilists! Much of the work of these travelling physicians was related to the wounds and injuries resulting from minor wars between city-states. *Epidemics* contains many descriptions of attending to catapult and sling wounds, and removing broken javelin and arrow-heads. Warfare thus afforded the opportunity to

develop surgical skills, but because standing armies were virtually unknown in the Hellenistic (Greek) world there was no opportunity for a physician to obtain permanent employment in the military.

Another major part of the physician's work was the repair of fractures. The traction apparatus required for the treatment of fractures was heavy and elaborate (see Figure 2.4), and as it would have been difficult to carry around it is likely that the places visited by physicians would have in residence an early form of surgical-appliance maker tending such equipment, on whom physicians would be dependent during their visits. In passing it is interesting to note that warfare and violence still act as a spur to innovation in health care. The management of chest and head wounds has made notable advances in the hospitals of Belfast since the 'troubles' that began in the 1960s.

Although the travelling tradition continued, cities began to appoint salaried physicians, funded by an annual tax. Such doctors were appointed to serve the poor, but were allowed to engage in private practice with the rich.

Fractures and traumatic surgery* apart, Greek physicians probably had little to offer in the way of effective

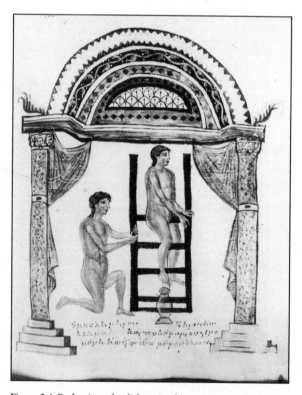

Figure 2.4 Reduction of a dislocation by traction apparatus.

*Surgery for the repair of injuries (traumas).

treatment for most of the illness they encountered. They did, however, offer two other services apart from the 'curing' of disease. The first was that of promoting good health. Physicians would prescribe a way of life which would help people to maintain their health. Such a regimen for health stressed diet, rest, and athletic competition — the last being an aspect of Greek life which was drawn on at the end of the nineteenth century with the revival of the Olympic Games.

The other activity that made up the work of physicians has been described by E.O. Phillips, a Belfast historian:

> Though they understood so little of the causes of disease, the Hippocratics had a good notion of the treatment of patients in such matters as rest and comfort, washing and warming, feeding with slops and drinks to keep up the strength, and on the psychological side, too, of the sympathy and encouragement needed to keep up trust and hope. (Phillips, 1973, p.75)

□ Make a short list of the physician's tasks mentioned in this passage. What formal occupational group would have most responsibility for these tasks in contemporary health care?

■ The tasks mentioned — washing, warming, feeding, comforting, encouraging, rehabilitating — form the stock in trade of modern nursing care.

The nurse did not exist in Greek medicine, and it was part of the job of the physician, or more likely the physician's assistant, along with lay carers, to provide what would now be considered nursing care.

The exception to this was the availability of midwives and wet-nurses for infants. Directions for choosing a wet-nurse appeared in the *Midwives Catechism*, a kind of Hippocratic 'Reader's Digest' handbook condensed from the gynaecology volumes of the *Hippocratic Corpus*:

> The wet-nurse should not be younger than twenty or older than forty. She must already have borne two or three children, be healthy, strong, plump and blooming; her breasts should be normal, relaxed, soft and unwrinkled, the nipples neither too large nor too small, too hard or too spongy; she must be even-tempered, charming, gentle ... her milk must be of just the right kind ... (Cited in Phillips, 1973, pp.166–7)

□ How would you summarise the kind of qualifications listed?

■ They are essentially a list of physiological, biological and personal attributes, rather than skills that had formally to be studied and learnt.

Wet-nursing was clearly, for biological reasons, women's work. However, as formal nursing expanded its role, it too remained almost exclusively women's work. Some of the reasons for this will emerge during the next two chapters. Meanwhile it is important to note that even as early as 400 BC, gender differences in health care occupations existed.

For all the various functions that physicians performed in ancient Greece, there was little specialisation,* such as between medicine and surgery. In general the *narrower* the skills of a physician the lower the esteem in which he was held. This is in contrast to today, when specialists are held in higher regard than generalists. Given the power and influence that physicians were gaining, it became necessary for some form of control or check on their activities and behaviour. The physicians themselves had drawn up, in the *Hippocratic Corpus*, many general and specific injunctions about their own deportment and behaviour. Some of these delineate the equivalent of 'bedside manner':

> The physician should have as good a colour and plumpness as nature intended, for most people think that a man in poor condition will not take good care of others. He should be clean in person, well-dressed and anointed with sweet-smelling unguents that arouse no suspicion ... In the expression of his face let him be gravely thoughtful but not harsh, for then he will appear to be arrogant and unkind ... Patients put themselves into the hands of their physicians, and at every moment he meets women, maidens and possessions very precious indeed, towards which he must use self-control. (Cited in Phillips, 1973, p.117)

Other instructions concern the crucial topic of payment for services:

> There should be no discussion of fees during the illness, for that will suggest that you will leave the patient if no agreement is reached, or at least neglect to propose immediate treatment. Such a worry will be harmful to the patient, particularly if the disease is acute. It is better to reproach a patient whom you have saved than to extort money from a man mortally sick. (Cited in Phillips, 1973, p.119)

□ This attitude towards payment suggests that a physician's income from practice might be irregular or unreliable. What might this imply about the social background of medical men?

---

*The meaning of the words 'physician' and 'medicine' has altered over the years. Nowadays 'physician' refers exclusively to a hospital doctor who specialises in the medical treatment of adults, as distinct from surgeons, psychiatrists, obstetricians and paediatricians. 'Medicine' refers both to the work of all types of doctor (e.g. medical practice) and specifically to the work of physicians (e.g. medical treatment, using drugs and other non-surgical procedures).

■ You have already seen that their esteem and respect was seen to depend in part on their being well dressed, well fed, etc. It seems likely, therefore, that they would have had to have come from a reasonably wealthy background, both to sustain their education and to give material support to their career.

While such regulation of physicians' behaviour by other physicians (so-called '*internal* rules of conduct') was regarded as acceptable for such matters as demeanour, what should happen if a physician, through obvious incompetence, injured or killed patients? And what should be done about people who pretended to be trained physicians? Could physicians be left to regulate fellow members of the occupation on such matters? Despite the apparent need for *external* rules of conduct, or laws, to cover such life and death issues, no legal regulations in fact existed to cover medical practise. The argument against such externally imposed discipline, and against any form of legal *licence* to practise, was put by Plato:

> that the status of a physician derived from his practice of medicine, that good ones would have higher status and bad ones lower, and that a legal licence would have to be sanctioned by politicians, who had no expertise in assessing competence to practice medicine. (Cited in Phillips, 1973, p.191)

□ What would you consider to be the most important assumption underpinning the argument that the social status or esteem of individual physicians derived from the quality of their practice of medicine?
■ The argument relies on the assumption that the public have access to sufficient information to assess the quality of care provided by a physician.

While ideally this may be desirable, in practice the lack of any external rules of conduct offers the public little protection against incompetent physicians.

Greek medicine was not only concerned with the health of individuals. The awareness of the importance of public health can be judged by the considerable weight that Hippocratic medicine placed on the proper balance between human beings and their environment. The Hippocratic treatise *Airs, Waters and Places* is the first known systematic treatment of environmental influences on health and for more than 2 000 years was the basic western epidemiological text. It distinguished between endemic and epidemic diseases and argued that endemic diseases were the product of an imbalance in the following five factors: climate, soil, water, mode of life and nutrition. In doing so, it served not only the practice of the travelling Greek physicians, but the interests of the Greek colonists. The treatise advises that before a settlement is decided upon physicians should be questioned and the character of the soil subjected to detailed investigation.

The extent to which such knowledge was put into practice can be judged by surviving examples of water supplies and sanitation. Pergamum, a Greek city-state in what is now Turkey, had by 200 BC an aqueduct installed on pure hydraulic principles. The source of water supply was a high-level reservoir at a height of about 1 220 feet on Mount Hagios Georgios, from which water was carried over intervening lower ground to a cistern 369 feet above sea-level. It is the finest of all the Greek water systems which now survives. Such systems had been used by the Greeks for many centuries. At some point in the sixth century BC Athens arranged for water to be piped from the hills ten miles away and, like all the Greek city-states, it had public officials, the *astynomi*, who were responsible for drainage and water-supply.

Here we may note that Aesculapius, the god of healing, had rivals: 'Hygiene is the modern ersatz for the cult of Hygeia, the lovely goddess who once watched over the health of Athens … [she] symbolized the virtues of a sane life in a pleasant environment'. But 'she never truly touched the hearts of the people' — Aesculapius was ascendant, and 'soon Hygeia was relegated to the role of a member of his retinue, usually as his daughter, sometimes as his sister or wife, but always subservient to him'. Even her sister, Panakeia, became more popular as a healing goddess, and 'her cult is alive today in the universal search for a panacea' (Dubos, 1979, p.7). Was Hygeia's demotion reflected in the status of the *astynomi* compared with the Hippocratic physicians? We can only speculate.

In the fourth century BC the Greeks, who had already colonised large areas of the Mediterranean, extended their empire into the Middle East, Egypt, and even reached northern India. Alexandria on the Mediterranean coast of Egypt became a great city during this period, and Greeks spread as settlers throughout this vastly expanded territory. With them went their physicians and medical ideas. With them also went armies, which increasingly employed physicians as salaried servants in garrisons, camps, and on campaigns. This expansion of the Hellenistic world led to confrontations with different religious systems, a factor that was to play an important part in the development not only of medicine but also education and employment.

□ Up to this period Greek religion and morality — although containing no influential priesthood — regarded the dead bodies of humans as sacred and did not permit the practice of dissection. What consequences do you think this had for Greek medicine?
■ It was a significant handicap to the furtherance of anatomical knowledge and teaching.

The Greek conquests threw existing religious systems into a melting pot. As a result of these religious changes restrictions on dissection were swept away, and it was this, more than anything, that guaranteed the power and success of the medical school in Alexandria, set up by Ptolemy the First (King of Egypt and former general of Alexander the Great), in the newly-founded Royal Academy or 'Museum' around 300 BC. To the Alexandrian school of medicine went leading physicians of the period, and from it were drawn physicians to work all over the Hellenistic world, and increasingly for the new Mediterranean power — Rome.

Rome — organisation and empire

The Roman city-state was in certain key respects far more military than the Greek city-states; indeed, the word '*populus*', from which the English word 'population' derives, originally meant a mass of infantry. Alexander's death in 323 BC marked the beginning of a long period of internal warfare in the Greek Empire, weakening the power of the city-states and allowing the Romans to enlarge and consolidate their power. In large part this resulted from the absorption of many Greek ideas, practices, skills and arts though to these the Romans added their interest in law and their brilliance as engineers. By the first century BC the Roman Empire was largely in control of the Hellenistic world and was beginning to expand beyond this. For the next three centuries its rule extended across most of Europe, North Africa, and west Asia.

Roman medicine was in many ways a direct continuation of Greek medicine, with the important difference that it was more militarised and more territorially diffused. Each legion of the Roman Army (between two and six thousand men) contained several physicians, designated as surgeons. Their relatively low rank indicates a lowly status more akin to tradesmen than general physicians. But they took their skills far and wide, even to the north-west fringes of the Roman Empire in north Britain, where in Hadrian's Wall there still sits a gravestone of a surgeon (Figure 2.5).

The Alexandrian school continued to be a major influence. More than 400 years after it was established it was to Alexandria that the Greek Galen — the most famous physician of the Roman Empire — travelled to study dissection, around AD 160. In contrast to Greek practice, the profession of medicine was a low-status occupation. Opulent Romans would commonly have as part of their establishment slaves who had been trained in medicine at their owner's expense. However, Greek physicians began to migrate — or be taken as slaves — to Rome in the third century BC and were soon much sought after. The status of the occupation began to rise from slave to 'freedman'. Only the rich could afford their services; the poor still relied on lay care and the gods, a fact that serves to remind us that natural medicine was only the tip of an essentially supernatural/magical iceberg of health care practices.

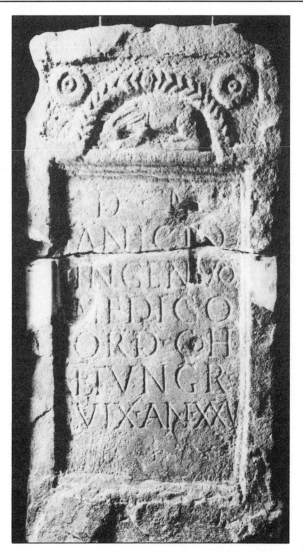

Figure 2.5 Third-century AD gravestone near Housesteads on Hadrians Wall, found in 1813: 'To the Spirits of the Departed and to Anicus Ingenuus, Medicus Ordinarius of the 1st Cohort of Tungrians, who lived 25 years'. The Tungrian legion drew recruits from Tungria, an area of modern Belgium.

The influx of the Greeks was not always welcomed:

All the dregs of Greece are pouring into our city … Language teacher, rhetorician, painter, masseur, surveyor, rope-dancer, soothsayer, magician, doctor. Nothing your hungry Greek can't do. (Juvenal, *Satires* III; cited in Christ, 1984, p.77)

But for all their scorn, the Romans did little to further Greek medical theory. Their strength lay instead in their systematic organisation. It was in Rome that the hospital first began to develop in Europe, principally with respect to the army, but also amongst private practitioners. Excavations at Pompeii suggest that some private doctors ran institutions somewhat like a modern convalescent or nursing home. Moreover, in the heyday of the empire in the first century AD, when it had around 60 million subjects, hospitals or infirmaries for slaves were also developed as part of a public medical service aimed specifically at the poor. In about AD 160 it was decreed that large cities should have ten municipal physicians, medium-sized towns, seven and small towns, five. The salaries of these *archiatri* were paid by the town council, but they were also allowed to accept fees from richer patients. An edict instructed them to:

> Think of them (the poor) rather than the rich; and where there is a question of fees, take as your reward, not what men fearing for their lives will promise, but what men recovering from illness will offer. (Cited in Simon, 1890, p.28)

Such measures, were part of a much wider shift in Roman social policy that took place in the first and second centuries AD. The acceptance, by town and city councils, of some of the responsibility for the health of the inhabitants led to their involvement in various public health measures. It was in this area that Rome made its mark, far outstripping the Greeks in engineering feats. The Greek geographer, Strabo, described the Rome of Emperor Tiberius (AD 14–37):

> Their underground sewers, with vaults of jointed stones, would in many places allow entire hay carts to drive through them. The quantities of water brought into the city are so large that whole rivers stream through the city and its underground drains, and that almost every house has water cisterns and piped water and abundantly spouting fountains. (Cited in Christ, 1984, p.148)

So important indeed were fresh water and adequate drainage to the Romans that the posts of *curator aquarum* (manager of the metropolitan water supply) and *curator alvi Tiberis et riparum et cloacarum urbis* (controller of the basin of the River Tiber, and of its embankments and of sewers) were amongst the most prestigious posts in the state, equivalent to that of governor of a province and only open to senators who had already served as consuls, the highest office of state.

The first great Roman aqueduct, the *Aqua Appia*, was built in 312 BC and eventually there were thirteen such aqueducts serving a population in Rome which various estimates place between 500 000 and one million. According to one estimate, the principal aqueducts delivered about forty gallons per head per day — a figure which still compares well with many modern cities. And, though

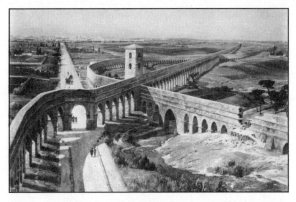

Figure 2.6 The aqueducts of Rome. This 'spaghetti junction' on the city outskirts is a remnant of over 30 miles of raised aqueduct in the 250 miles of channel and tunnel bringing water to the imperial capital. (From a painting by Zeno Diemer, Deutches Museum, Munich.)

Rome itself had the most splendid of all such aqueducts, similar constructions were used throughout the Empire — the remains of no fewer than 200 still survive across Europe, the Near East and North Africa (Figure 2.6).

Public latrines were in general use, at least for men, and though some involved a small charge others were probably free. Some of these undoubtedly discharged into the sewers and some had a water service by which their contents were actually flushed out. Public latrines at Ostia, still existing today, reflect the pride the Romans had in their sanitary facilities as well as their very different attitudes towards privacy — they had marble seats that could accommodate thirty people at a time.

Responsibility for building the larger drainage schemes in Rome, such as the aqueducts and the elaborate sewers, rested with the senate and 'censors', the ruling class of Rome. Such schemes were often dependent on the donations of the wealthiest citizens — an action that could be employed as an election gambit by the donor. Public health measures also included banning the casting of filth into the common way, forbidding burial within the city walls, and ensuring that house builders left at least two and a half feet width of land between buildings. In addition, the *Aediles*, who administered each of the four districts of the city of Rome, were responsible for the efficient repair of the network of drains, public buildings and places, proper cleansing and paving of streets, preventing the nuisances of dangerous buildings and animals and foul smells, supplying the market of the capital with good and cheap grain, destroying unsound goods and overseeing baths, taverns and brothels.

Roman civic engineering was also concerned with personal hygiene. Public baths with hot and cold water — the *thermae* — were available to everyone who was a citizen of Rome — however, slaves (perhaps 50 per cent of the population) were excluded. At Rome's height a thousand such public baths existed. Attached to these thermae were gymnasia and other facilities. Not surprisingly, Rome also had a soap factory.

There were, then, many ways in which the Romans acknowledged at least in part, the Roman saying '*Salus publica supremo lex*' (public health is the supreme law). However, there were some areas left untouched, despite the health hazards being recognised. Martial mentions the diseases peculiar to sulphur workers; Lucretius refers to the hard lot of gold miners; and Galen commented that:

> the life of many men is involved in the business of their occupation and it is inevitable that they should be harmed by what they do and that it should be impossible to change it. (Cited in Brockington, 1975, p.118)

We are rightly impressed by the engineering achievements of the Romans, their water supplies, sewers and baths. But what *effect* did it have on health, and, if it was effective, how many people actually benefited? One history text summarises the known information on this as follows:

> the evidence is scanty and derived in the main from funeral inscriptions and '*stelae*'. The sample of the Roman population for which we have information is very far from random, and is, by and large, composed of those who were wealthy enough to record their lifespan. The average age at death for adults appears to have been between thirty and thirty-five years. One assumes that there was a high rate of infant mortality, and the average expectation of life at birth was probably not a great deal more than twenty years. (Pounds, 1974, p.7)

This is the picture among the better-off Roman citizens. As we have already suggested some groups didn't receive all the privileges of Roman citizenship. Rome had major slums where the poor and slaves lived, and behind the hygienic façade of Rome, were slaves, subject to many ills and occupied day and night in the baths oiling and caring for their masters. Some writings testify to the conditions under which the poor lived, telling, for example, of the terrible noises of collapsing buildings and the constant hazards of fire from timber buildings and oil lamps.

Moreover, it must be remembered that Rome was an exception, an urban island in an ocean of rural life. Rome lived off the land, extracting the land's surplus and keeping the great majority of the Empire's population at subsistence level by taxation and rent. And it contributed little in return, for Rome was not a centre of manufacturing or industry. In fact productive labour was held in contempt, as fit only for slaves: 'slavery' and 'labour' were interchangeable words. 'Dying slavery left behind its poisonous sting by branding as ignoble the work of the free. This was the blind alley in which the Roman world was caught', wrote a later observer, Friedrich Engels. The upkeep of the massive infrastructure of public health and civic buildings became an increasing burden. On top of these problems, a 'plague', perhaps smallpox, swept through the Empire in AD 165–180 and again in AD 251–66. At the peak of the latter outbreak, 5 000 people were said to have died each day in Rome. The social institution that would dominate health care for the next 1 000 years — the Christian church — took strength from these weaknesses. It recruited amongst urban slaves, and preached a message of religious duty towards the poor. It preached the dignity of manual labour. And in the face of random deaths from epidemics, it preached a life after death, a means to cope with the pervasive uncertainties of disease.

The fall of Rome, the rise of the Church

The Romans' European empire collapsed in the fourth and fifth centuries AD under the weight of successive barbarian invasions of Germanic peoples. With Rome gone, the Graeco-Roman health tradition, its scientific interests, its learning and its achievements in public health, largely disappeared from western Europe for many centuries. In AD 537 the eleven principal aqueducts still supplying Rome were destroyed during a siege by the Goths, and Rome itself was devastated. Pope Adrian the First undertook their partial restoration in AD 776, but they were then, like Rome itself, merely a shadow of their former glory.

Health care traditions based fundamentally on magic and religion became wellnigh ubiquitous. One such example is *The Leechbook of Bald* (*c.* AD 900–950), a medical text introduced to Britain by Germanic settlers, and the most important Saxon medical work to survive. Although it has some classical influences relating back to Rome, it also contains, for example, advice on methods for combating the harmful influence of elves. Physicians were defined often by the most incidental criteria, as is apparent from one Norse saga which records that in 1043, when King Magnus the Good found that after the Battle of Lyrskop Heath there were insufficient doctors to attend all the casualties; he simply selected those:

> who had the softest hands and told them to bind the wounds of the people, and although none of them had ever tried it before, they all afterwards became the best of doctors (from whom) many good doctors are descended. (Cited in Rubin, 1974, pp.102–3)

None the less, though Rome itself had succumbed to the invaders, Roman influence lived on. A major eastern part of the Empire, centred on Byzantium, and practising Christianity, survived intact another 1 000 years. Major

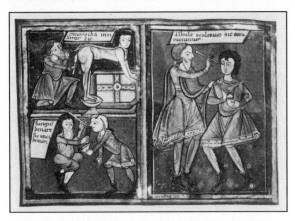

Figure 2.7 Anglo-Saxon surgery. Twelfth-century doctors, or *leeches*, undertook a number of surgical procedures. The illustration shows surgery for haemorrhoids, with the buttocks held open by a retractor; for a nasal polyp, with the patient holding a bowl to collect blood draining from his nose; and for a cataract of the eye. *The Leechbook of Bald*, and other texts of the period, suggest more treatments for eye conditions than any other single malady. Eye disorders probably arose from vitamin A deficiency in the diet, and from smoky and unhygienic living conditions.

aspects of Graeco-Roman civilisation were also inherited by cultures outside Europe.

The Eastern Empire carried on some of the old traditions of Rome, while others were radically transformed. In AD 312, Emperor Constantine had been converted to Christianity, which then became the official religion of the Empire. Caring and healing, activities central to Christian teaching, were therefore very much part of religious work. The Council of Nicaea (AD 325) instructed bishops to establish a hospital in every city that had a cathedral. An early example was that created (between AD 369 and 372) by St Basil at Caesarea in ancient Palestine. The hospital comprised several sections dealing with different classes of ailment; the physicians lived on the premises; and it cared not only for the sick and the infirm, but also travellers and the very poor.

☐ In what way is this unlike a modern hospital?

■ The modern hospital caters only for the sick and for certain sorts of infirmity. Travellers and the very poor are cared for in other ways, for example, in hotels and hostels.

Although the function of hospitals has shifted from simply providing hospitality to providing health care, it is important to note that even in the 1980s a large proportion of hospital beds in Britain serve as a means of caring for rather than 'treating' people. This is true for many of those who are infirm, mentally ill, mentally handicapped, and physically disabled.

The relative complexity of a Byzantine hospital was sketched in the introductory chapter, and as you will see shortly, the hospitals and health care of the Islamic world, China, and India were also sophisticated. Despite the spread of Christianity through western Europe, nothing as sophisticated was to appear there for a long time. Instead, a different version of the hospital emerged, based on monasteries with monks and nuns tending the sick and the poor. Not every religious order contributed; indeed, Cistercian monks were not allowed to buy drugs, take medicines or visit doctors themselves, nor were the Carthusians. But the Augustinians made a special point of caring for the sick and the poor and some monastic physicians and surgeons rose to positions of great influence. Abbot Baldwin of Bury St Edmunds was physician to both Edward the Confessor and William the Conqueror. The earliest hospital in Britain is traditionally thought to have been St Peters at York, founded in 937, refounded in 1155 after a fire and by 1370 containing over 200 sick and infirm inmates. Indeed, by the middle of the fourteenth century, there were more than 600 hospitals in England, though many were small. An example of one which survives to the present day is the Lord Leycester Hospital in Warwick which still has its complement of twelve pensioners.

Similar developments had taken place on the Continent. Overall the estimate suggests that there were as many as 19 000 hospitals in Europe by the end of the thirteenth century.

In addition, there was a similar number of leprosaria (places for the confinement of lepers).* These institutions first appeared in the seventh century AD following the edict of the Council of Lyons in AD 573 which restricted the free association of lepers with healthy people. Lepers were outcasts, deprived of all their civic rights and declared socially dead long before their physical demise. Given such dreadful consequences, the diagnosis of someone as suffering from leprosy was clearly of vital importance. This decision was taken by a group including a bishop, other clerics, and a leper, who acted as a specialist on the subject. (There are parallels with the current interest in involving chronic sufferers and the disabled in decisions about their own treatment and about the development and provision of health services.)

Leprosy is a chronic bacterial infection causing peripheral nerve damage, loss of sensation, and muscle weakness, particularly in hands and feet. It is still widespread in tropical and sub-tropical regions of the world. It is described in more detail in The Open University (1985) *The Biology of Health and Disease*, The Open University Press, Chapter 14 (U205 *Health and Disease*, Book IV). Some possible reasons for its eventual disappearance from Europe are discussed in *The Health of Nations, ibid.*, Chapter 8 (U205 Book III).

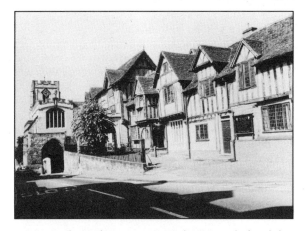

Figure 2.8 The Lord Leycester Hospital in Warwick, founded to provide accommodation for the poor. It is now inhabited by ex-servicemen and their wives.

□ What aspect of the medieval management of leprosy has had a lasting impact on the way infectious diseases are managed?
■ The methodical eradication of the disease by isolating and excluding sufferers from society.

What were medieval hospitals in western Europe like? Their organisation was largely determined by their key function, which was not the care of the sick, but rather the service of God. Beds were situated in the naves of churches — partly because this was the largest space available, but also so that the sick could see the altar. Indeed, it was the duty of the inmates to spend their time in hospital praying for the souls of others — particularly for that of the institution's founder. Whereas the hospitals of Byzantium often made elaborate provision for both professional medical care as well as prayer, the medieval hospitals of the west lacked specific provision for the former — the Savoy was the first London hospital to be regularly attended by professional surgeons and physicians, but that was not until 1515.

In principle, hospital care was free. Practice, however, could be rather different. Elderly people no longer able to manage without help might make over their property to hospitals in return for the promise of aid, and some hospitals did charge fees — a practice which was regularly condemned but still continued. However, such payment never represented more than a small fraction of the running costs. How was it then, that the Church could administer a service that extended to 19 000 institutions?

□ What explanations can you suggest?
■ There appear to be two possibilities:
1 Care was provided by monks and nuns who would not have expected or received financial rewards;
2 The Church was wealthy enough to be able to afford to provide hospital care.

In fact, records from medieval times show that the Church was indeed very wealthy. By the end of the seventh century it is estimated that one third of the productive land of France was in Church hands. In England the great build-up of Church lands occurred during the period *c*. AD 600–1100. Analysis of the 'Domesday Book', the land survey of the conquering Norman aristocracy compiled in 1086, suggests that the Church then owned 26 per cent of all rural property in England.

How had the Church gained the wealth which enabled it to fund its elaborate system of health care? Part of the answer lies in the religious beliefs of the period. Good works, so it was held, enabled those who performed them to gain salvation and to avoid undue pain and suffering in Purgatory. Charity towards the poor and needy speeded the souls of the rich towards heaven. And after the fall of Rome, with the whole of western Europe plunged into a state of flux for hundreds of years, the only institution providing stability was the Church. Right across Europe, monasteries were run on similar lines; they fulfilled similar roles in relation to healing and medicine and were often run by like-minded people speaking the same international language (Latin) and educated in the same centres of learning. Europe might consist of a myriad kingdoms and fiefdoms, secular (non-religious) power might change hands, and epidemics and poor harvests might devastate the population, but amidst all this vicissitude and uncertainty stood the security of the Church. Thus, the Church could be viewed as a passive recipient of wealth donated by individuals out of a sense of gratitude for the spiritual as well as physical shelter it provided. However, this ignores the possibility of the Church playing a more active role in achieving its position of vast wealth and power. An explanation of how this could have been achieved has been suggested by an anthropologist, Jack Goody.

He points out that in pre-Christian Europe forms of clan organisation existed in which property belonged not just to the individual but to the family. Therefore, there was a whole series of devices to ensure that the clan maintained its grip on the property that its members had acquired over generations: for example, by heir adoption, or by restricting bequests to institutions.

According to Goody, all this was to be changed by the Christian church. By the fourth century it had been granted the special privilege of receiving bequests from the faithful. Thereafter, many traditional forms of marriage were forbidden as incestuous, the offspring of concubinage were defined as illegitimate and unable to inherit, and adoption disappeared (it did not return to England until 1926). These changes led to the huge and rapid increase in the Church's wealth and power. A French poet in about 1200 wrote:

> Today when a man falls ill and lies down to die, he does not think of his sons or his nephews or cousins: he summons the Black Monks of St Benedict and gives them his lands, his revenues, his ovens and his mills. The men of this age are impoverished and the clerics are daily becoming richer. (Cited in Goody, 1983, p.105)

What effect might this huge accumulation of wealth by the Church have had on traditional patterns of caring? By providing funds for an elaborate system of hospitals, it may have reduced the ability of the clan or family to provide lay care for its members, while at the same time offering alternative ways of providing care.

Although the most striking fact about health care in this period from the sixth century AD onwards is the power and influence of the Church and its development of an elaborate system of hospitals, health care was not entirely dominated by the Church and its teachings. Many traditional practices continued in western Europe much as before, sometimes despite the Church's opposition. For example, fostering and wet-nursing were traditional amongst the Viking and Germanic peoples. Churchmen fulminated against them over the centuries, but their protests seem to have had little effect.

The key role played by the Church in the delivery of formal health care in the early medieval period has had a lasting impact on health care occupations and institutions.

☐ Can you suggest some influences that are still apparent today?

■ You may have thought of the names of hospitals such as St Bartholomew's, St Thomas', St Mary's and so on; the uniforms worn by nurses which were until recently, and still are in some places, modelled on a nun's habit; and the designation of senior nurses as 'Sister'.

This involvement of organised religion in health care still runs deep in many countries of the world, as you will see later in the book. However, around the end of the tenth century, a millenium on from the Christian church's origins, Europe began to change.

Secular developments in medieval health care

Throughout the Dark Ages the Church in Europe had indeed been an island of continuity in a sea of unstable backwardness and stagnation. India, China and the Islamic world all were more advanced in technology, science, armaments and medicine. But changes in Europe reversed this position, as stagnation and backwardness gave way to expansion and, eventually, dominance. Quite rapid population growth began, and this continued up to the great plagues of the mid-fourteenth century. Forests and fens were claimed for agriculture. A long construction boom began, not least affecting hospitals, monasteries and churches: 'so on the threshold of the aforesaid thousand year ... every nation of Christendom rivalled with the other, which should worship in the seemliest buildings. So it was as though the very world had shaken herself and cast off her old age, and were clothing herself everywhere in a white garment of churches' (Raoul Glaber, an eleventh-century monk; cited in Pounds, 1974, p.91). New technologies began to appear: in northern Italy the invention of a way of making perfectly clear glass led around 1280 to the invention in Tuscany of spectacles, thus offering for the first time in human history an effective way of overcoming the widespread disability of visual impairment. Among the poor, access to this invention was limited (indeed a sizeable unsatisfied need for spectacles still existed in 1948 when the National Health Service began in Britain). They spread rapidly amongst those who could afford them, however, and within 60 years of their invention the Florentine scholar, Petrarch, was boasting that he didn't use them, thereby implying that most of his acquaintances did.

What was at the root of this profound change across Europe? It seems likely that the answer has something to do with the growth of urban centres; towns, moreover, which were not in the hands of aristocrats, officials and landed gentry, as in the past and elsewhere in the world, but rather had become 'dominated, politically, socially, and culturally by the merchants and the moneychangers ... and also by the pharmacists, the notaries, the lawyers, the judges, the doctors and the like' (Cipolla, 1976a, p.18). These were the *burghers*, and their position of power, propelled by their commercial interests, began the transformation of Europe. Around the tenth and eleventh centuries there were hardly more than 100 places in Europe that could claim to be towns: by the end of the fifteenth century there were four to five *thousand*. The burghers, merchants and their towns now began to move to centre stage in the provision of health care, slowly displacing the Church and eventually secularising health care.

The changes beginning to transform Europe spread outwards from Italy, and can be traced through the rise of the first European medical school in the town of Salerno, 35 miles south of Naples. According to legend it had been founded in the ninth century by a Jew, an Arab, a Greek and a Latin, but whatever its origins, its real influence dates from the end of the eleventh century. People came to be trained there from all over Europe and its position in the Mediterranean gave it access to Jewish writers and Arabic medical learning which had, partly via Byzantium, inherited the Graeco-Roman tradition.

The medical course at Salerno lasted five years. The influence of the church was still present in that anatomy teaching excluded human dissection. Instead the anatomy of the pig was studied — *Anatomia Porci* by Kapho was the first European textbook of anatomy. After five years students did one year of practical work under supervision and were awarded a degree, after which they were entitled to call themselves 'Magister' or 'Doctor' — it was in Salerno that the title 'doctor' was used for the first time.

Following the example of Salerno, the thirteenth century saw further medical schools created in nearby Naples and in the new universities of Montpellier, Bologna, Padua, Paris, Oxford and Cambridge. As the number of university-trained doctors expanded so the Church began to withdraw from at least part of the growing medical market. Hospitals continued to be based in churches, but the practice of medicine in the monasteries was gradually stopped and when hospitals wished to have a physician or a surgeon they began to call on the new university-trained doctors. In 1139, worried about monks turning their medical knowledge to personal profit, Pope Innocent prohibited the clergy from any further study of medicine. This ban was clearly not that effective, for in 1215 Pope Innocent III produced a modified version of the earlier ruling, this time barring monks from performing any surgery which involved the shedding of blood. Again, the new ban was not immediately effective — the surgeon to the King of England from 1233 to 1254 was a monk. Nevertheless, gradually the training and practice of medicine became a *secular* rather than a religious affair.

☐ The secularisation of medicine meant that some people who had previously not had access to training, could now study to be physicians. Which people were these?

■ Women.

By all known measures of mortality or life-expectancy, medieval women were much worse off than men. But in the twelfth, and particularly the thirteenth century their social standing improved: one sign of this was the suddenly elevated importance of the Virgin Mary in Christian symbolism and art. Women had access to the medical school in Salerno, as is shown by the case of the eleventh-century practitioner, Trotula, who turned her training to account by producing a treatise on obstetrics and gynaecology:

Because there are many women who have numerous diverse illnesses — some of them almost fatal — and because they are also ashamed to reveal and tell their distress to any man, I therefore shall write somewhat to cure their illnesses ... to help their secret maladies so that one woman may aid another in her illness and not divulge her secrets to such discourteous men.

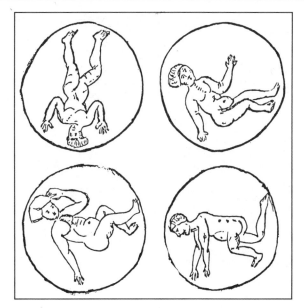

Figure 2.9 These four figures come from an early fifteenth-century treatise on obstetrics and gynaecology, part of which is ascribed to Trotula, and other parts to the second-century AD writings of Soranus of Ephesus. The treatise contains sixteen such figures showing unnatural birth positions the midwife is to correct; for example, when both hands are extended 'she should put his hands to his sides, take the child's head, and gently bring him forth' (Rowland, 1981, p. 59). Figures drawn from the originals by Edna G. Murphy.

(Translation into modern English from an early fifteenth-century English manuscript, ascribed to Trotula (Rowland, 1981, p.59))

Some illustrations from Trotula's manual are reproduced in Figure 2.9.

The names of a few early English women practitioners are also known. They include Matilda 'la leche' (the leech) from Wallingford *c*. 1232 and Katherine 'la surgiene' *c*. 1286, whose father and brother were also surgeons. Since medical practice was often a family business, husbands, wives, sons and daughters might all engage in the trade.

However, though women did clearly play a role in the healing trades, there were persistent, diverse attempts to drive them out by male practitioners. For example, Latin, an essential part of the training, ceased to be taught in nunneries by the fourteenth century and women had no access to the new grammar schools. At the same time, the new profession of medicine developed trade-associations or guilds and tried to bar from practice all those who had no formal qualifications. In 1421 the London physicians petitioned the Privy Council to ban women from the trade — though this attempt did not succeed. On the Continent, where the guild structure was more developed, such efforts

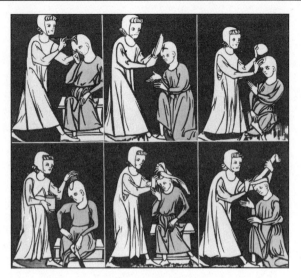

Figure 2.10 The surgeon (is it perhaps *la surgienne*?) in this series of thirteenth-century illustrations appears to be conducting a form of the operation known as *trepanning* or *trephining*, which consists in making perforations in the skull and removing disks of bone. From the evidence of excavated skulls, the operation was performed by Neolithic surgeons, and is still encountered in parts of the world. It was common in Europe until the nineteenth century: thirty-two trephinations being carried out in St George's and Guy's Hospitals in London between 1870 and 1877, for example. The reasons for the operation are unclear; it may have been to allow the escape of demons and evil spirits, or to relieve cranial compression in cases of injury. From a treatise on surgery in the British Museum.

were more successful. For example, in 1484 in Paris all women, except the widows of surgeons, lost the right to practise surgery. Despite such bans, female practitioners still continued in practice. None the less, they were largely excluded from the more lucrative aspects of medical work.

At the same time as the practice of medicine was becoming increasingly secularised, so too the administrative control of hospitals throughout western Europe was undergoing an important shift towards much greater secular involvement. Monks and nuns still staffed the hospitals, which remained fundamentally religious institutions, but the ever more powerful merchants increasingly financed or came to control the motley array of hospitals and alms houses. Wealthy guilds of merchants might set up their own hospital and individuals who were particularly well-off might even create their own foundation. Monarchs too took a hand in all this — the inmates of the Savoy hospital had dressing-gowns which bore the Tudor livery, as did the counterpanes on their beds — there was to be no mistaking just who was their benefactor.

Aside from the growing wealth of the merchants and towns, one other factor led to the increase in secular involvement with the management of the hospitals, namely the administrative and financial incompetence of many of those who ran them. Hospitals were often the subject of considerable scandal. Many of the problems were due to the highly insecure nature of hospital finances. While some hospitals were richly endowed, others were heavily dependent on public charity and where this faltered, those who ran them had to look to other ways of raising money: these included turning a hospital into a school and neglecting the aged inmates; substituting the provision of meals by tokens which could be exchanged for food from private vendors; and maltreating the staff of monks and nuns. An inquiry in 1431 at St Mary's Bishopsgate in London revealed that the seven sisters who worked there were grossly overworked and deprived of adequate food and clothing. And inquiry after inquiry had to remind brothers and sisters of their sacred duty to tend the sick (Rawcliffe, 1984).

Secularisation of health care in the late medieval period did little to alter the different types of care and welfare that people of different backgrounds received. This is well illustrated by the way the mentally retarded and mentally ill were treated. In 1247 the first hospital in England for the care of the insane was founded in London — St Mary's Bethleham, which later became known as 'Bedlam' (Figure 2.11).

This hospital was concerned primarily with the care of the poor. For well-off members of society there were other provisions. As the American historian Richard Neugebauer (1978) has shown, from at least the thirteenth century, the English Crown claimed various rights over the property of both those who were considered to be 'natural fools' (mentally retarded) and those '*non compos mentis*' (the latter term was replaced by 'lunatic' in the fifteenth century). The King was entitled to the revenues of the lands and possessions of 'natural fools' during their lifetime and, in return, was obliged to protect and support them, though not their families. As for the '*non compos mentis*', the King had no claim on their estates, but was expected to ensure that both they and their families did not suffer by reason of insanity. Thus, an insane Earl would be maintained in the style of an Earl, a Baron in the style of a Baron. To what extent such royal responsibilities for the maintenance of both the retarded and the insane were prompted by financial benefits for the Crown is not clear. It was certainly an important device for raising money for the monarch.

The burghers' increasingly active interest and role in maintaining the hospitals and other institutions extended into the field of public health. Although the great civil engineering works of the Romans were not to be repeated until the eighteenth and nineteenth centuries in Europe, many other measures were instituted during the late medieval period to improve and protect the health of the new urban populations. These took three forms: (a) the

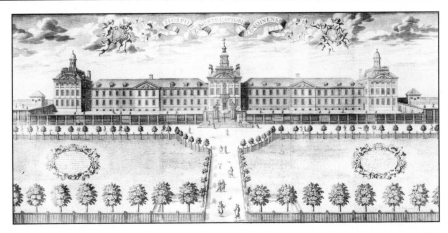

Figure 2.11 Bedlam. The first Bethlem was in Bishopsgate. In 1676 this was left for a site in Moorfields, shown here in an engraving by R. White: this was the *Bedlam* of the eighteenth century. In 1815 another move took Bethlem Royal Hospital to St George's Fields, Southwark. This last building is now the Imperial War Museum, the current Bethlem Hospital being in Beckenham, Kent.

creation of administrative measures to control the spread of disease; (b) efforts to deal with the sanitary problems of urban life; and (c) the provision of health care and social assistance to at least some of the poor and the destitute.

A succession of statutes in England attempting to confine the poor to their parish and restrict the number of wandering tramps and vagabonds was instituted in 1348 with the arrival of the Black Death. Another administrative measure, first introduced in Venice, was that of *quarantine* (from the Italian '*quaranta*' meaning 'forty') — the period of forty days during which a ship arriving in port was allowed no contact with the shore. Venice, a thriving seaport trading with the East, was particularly vulnerable to the spread of epidemic diseases such as the plague and appears to have taken a lead in establishing public hygiene regulations and enforcing strict quarantine on ships during the fourteenth century.

Despite such measures, infectious diseases repeatedly swept across Europe. In Italy, a major institution in the public health organisation of all towns was the *lazaretto* or pest-house. This was a building, often outside the walls of the town, for isolating people thought to have or to be incubating an infection. Although Venice and Milan had permanent lazarettos by the fifteenth century, most towns made temporary use of other buildings during an epidemic. As may be imagined, there was considerable resistance both on the part of patients and staff to being confined to such buildings (see Figure 3.1). The high mortality suffered by physicians led some to suggest that the patients should be 'cured at a distance' by shouting out their symptoms and history, and in reply the physician would shout out the treatment.

The rapid growth of population in towns in the late medieval period, combined with the need to contain people within the town or city walls led to increasing overcrowding. Although people switched from rural to urban living, they maintained many of the characteristics of rural life, such as keeping farm animals as a source of food. Towns had to introduce many regulations in an attempt to maintain and improve the health of their inhabitants. For example, in 1185 Paris became the first town to start paving the streets. In 1276, municipal slaughterhouses were introduced in Augsberg, while in 1281, pigs were forbidden in the streets of London. The last was followed by a whole series of regulations to restrict offensive trades: tallow-melting was no longer allowed in Chepe (an area of London); tailors were banned from scouring fur in daytime; the flaying of dead horses in the street was no longer allowed; and the solder-melting of plumbers in Eastcheap was made conditional upon raising the shaft of the furnace, presumably to alleviate the problems caused by smoke and fumes. Slaughtering of oxen, sheep, swine and other large animals was eventually banished from the city around 1370, and under Richard II in 1388 the first English general statute against nuisances near cities and towns was passed.

Increasingly from the fourteenth century on, town councils introduced water supplies. Some of the fountains that still exist in many European cities date back to the late medieval period when water supplies for the populace were being established.

Unlike the control of infections and sanitary regulations, social assistance for the relief of the poor remained largely a Church function throughout the medieval period. Since its earliest days, the clergy had distributed parochial funds to the poor parishioners. These funds were in a tradition that would be greatly elaborated in later centuries. It should not, however, be assumed that the provision of relief was generous. At its best it probably merely ensured survival. Nor should it be assumed that relief was freely available. Since the very earliest times philanthropy and charity have often sought to ensure that those receiving help are deserving of it. This ethos found its way into statutes as early as 1349 when under Edward III the giving of alms to 'valiant and sturdy beggars' was forbidden. Distinguishing between the 'deserving poor' — the old, the sick, the disabled — and the 'undeserving poor' — the lazy, the idle, the alcoholic — was to become a key feature of the debate on the Poor Laws in Tudor England, as you will see in the next chapter.

During the late medieval period, from 1000–1500, there were some notable achievements in the field of health care, many of which have left their mark up to the present day. George Rosen, a medical historian, is in no doubt about the impact this period had on the following centuries:

> These attempts to create a rational system of public hygiene are all the more impressive when one recalls that they were undertaken in a world in which superstition was rampant ... Most significant of all ... is the fact that in the medieval period were developed the basic patterns of thought and practice within which public health would function for the next two and a half centuries. (Rosen, 1958, p.80)

Europe and the world: early exchanges

Surveying the period covered by the chapter as a whole, perhaps the most significant aspect of the late medieval period was the changing status of Europe and European health care, relative to the rest of the world. We have already alluded to developments in India, China and the Islamic world. Let's now look briefly at the way European health care influenced and was influenced by this wider context, beginning with Vedic medicine in India.

Early Vedic medicine was magical and empirical. For example, sacred songs and rituals were used to ward off disease, but recourse was made to an extensive range of plant-based remedies. Magic and empiricism were not separate.* For example, magical rites involved animal sacrifice, and in consequence anatomical knowledge of sacrificial animals such as the horse was extensive. Around the sixth century BC, Vedic medical practice was systematically brought together in a codified body of knowledge and doctrine known as *Ayurveda*, or 'the science of life'. Ayurvedic medicine was in many ways similar to Greek medicine: its theoretical basis was a non-empirical model of bodily elements, or humours, that

caused illness if they became unbalanced. As with Greek medicine, some aspects of medical practice were highly developed.

☐ What was the main success of Greek medical practice?
■ The surgical treatment of wounds and lacerations largely as a consequence of the constant presence of warfare.

The same was true of Ayurvedic medicine. The closeness of Ayurvedic and Greek medicine may well have been reinforced in the fourth century BC, for in 334 BC Alexander embarked on his extensive campaign to extend Hellenistic influence. This took his armies as far as the River Indus (in modern-day Pakistan). It is reported that his armies employed Indian physicians. Although his empire broke up after his death in 323 BC, the campaign inaugurated a long period of trade between the Hellenistic world and India, which included the transfer of medical knowledge and health care practices.

Around the same time China was undergoing a fundamental change that was to affect Chinese, and eventually European, health care: Confucianism. Confucius was an aristocratic state official, whose primary concern was to lay out a system of government that would put an end to internal warring. It is within this canon of work that the classical Chinese system of medicine evolved, but the crucial point is that Confucianism is located within a different philosophical system, one that does not correspond to categories of western thought such as nature, anatomy, causation and diagnosis.

We know little about early Chinese medical science, and even less about the forms taken by medical practice and health care. What is not in doubt is that the Chinese civilisation of the Han dynasty was at least as powerful, populous, wealthy and sophisticated as the Roman Empire with which it tenuously traded around the second century AD. From the seventh to the thirteenth centuries AD China was without equal in the world.

The influence of Chinese medicine must be considered with some caution. As the Cambridge scholar, Christopher Cullen, has recently pointed out:

> Despite the mushrooming growth of literature devoted to Chinese medical science in recent years it must still be said that the amount of serious scholarship worth the name is relatively small so far as Western languages are concerned. (Cullen, 1983, p.490)

The Islamic contribution to the history of health care has often been under-estimated. In the sixth century AD the city of Gondeshapur near Baghdad began to grow rapidly as a centre of learning, attracting Greek, Syrian, Persian, Hindu

---

*Magic, empiricism and 'humours' are all discussed in *Medical Knowledge: Doubt and Certainty*, ibid. (U205 Book II).

and Jewish scholars. Here most Greek writing on medicine was translated into Syrian, Persian and the emerging lingua franca of Arabic. In the eighth century AD the Muslim rulers created and sustained the large hospital of Gondeshapur. In the ninth century a library was established in Baghdad with texts gathered from all over the Islamic empire and the Mediterranean. India also had a considerable impact on Islam — all chemists drew on Indian knowledge of transmutation and the properties of metals.

Foremost among Islamic scholars, and equal to any figure in medical history, was Abu Bakr Muhammad ibn Zakariya al-Razi, sometimes known by the latinised name Rhazes. His work took classical Greek and Indian writings as its starting point. His work in hospitals in Baghdad and elsewhere attached great importance to therapy and to observation. It was his emphasis on systematic observation that led him to make the first distinction between smallpox and measles.

What do we know of Islamic health care? From recent research by the American Islamic scholar, Emillie Savage-Smith, a picture emerges of an elaborate and sophisticated system of provision. At the beginning of the ninth century a hospital was opened in Baghdad modelled on the medical centre at Gondeshapur, marking the start of four centuries of hospital building throughout the Islamic world — from Spain in the west to Syria in the east (most is known about those built in Syria and Egypt in the twelfth and thirteenth centuries):

They were built on a cruciform plan with four central *iwans* or vaulted halls, with many adjacent rooms including kitchens, storage areas, a pharmacy, some living quarters for staff, and sometimes a library. Each iwan was usually provided with fountains to provide a supply of clean water. There was a separate hall for women patients ... There was also an area for surgical cases and a special ward for the mentally ill ... There frequently were out-patient clinics with a free dispensary of medicaments. The staff included pharmacists and a roster of physicians who were required at appointed times to be in attendance and make the rounds of patients, prescribing medications. These were assisted by stewards and orderlies as well as a considerable number of male and female attendants who tended the basic needs of the patients. (Savage-Smith, 1984, p.60)

☐ Of what other medical hospital should this remind you?
■ The description of the hospital in Constantinople in 1136.

In fact, the Islamic hospitals were similar to the Byzantine hospitals of earlier centuries, but built and run on a much larger scale. This is an example of how the Graeco-Roman traditions of Europe were taken over and maintained by Islam. There were other similarities between Christian Europe and the Islamic empire, as this quote illustrates:

All the hospitals in Islamic lands were financed from the revenues of a charitable trust called a *waqf*. Wealthy men and especially the rulers, donated property as an endowment whose revenue went towards building and maintaining the institution ... The income from the endowment would pay the maintenance and running costs of the hospital, and sometimes would supply a small stipend to the patient upon dismissal. (Savage-Smith, 1984, p.60)

☐ In what way was this similar to western Europe?
■ Income from church endowments were used to provide health care in much the same way.

The extent of the influence of the Islamic hospital system on later European hospital development is still largely unknown. The Islamic influence was felt directly in Spain, where Cordova and Granada became centres of western Islam, the latter being the site of the first Islamic hospital in Spain, constructed in 1397.

What is clear is that Islam exercised a decisive influence on the revival of learning in Europe after the tenth century. It was the Islamic libraries that preserved, translated, used and added to the classical literature of Greek medicine, philosophy and science, during the centuries when it had all but disappeared from Europe. The story of Constantine the African (1010–1087) illustrates this perfectly. After almost forty years of travelling round Arab centres of learning, he arrived at Salerno with a huge pile of Arabic manuscripts on medicine and retired to the monastery of Monte Casino to translate or retranslate them for use at the medical school, thereby fostering the revival of classic learning in medicine in late medieval Europe.

As to the independent impact of Islamic thought and science on Europe, it is necessary only to note the ousting of Roman numerals by the Arab numerical notation, and the introduction of such words as 'alchemy', 'algebra' and 'hazard'.

The influence of Islam was not only felt in Europe, but in India where, from the twelfth century onwards, western India came under direct Muslim rule. The system of medicine the Muslims brought to India was called *Unani*. There is an irony in the fact that Unani medicine is now regarded as 'traditional', in contrast to modern western medicine, for the word 'Unani' in fact means 'Greek'.

European health care, therefore, was involved in a much wider international exchange of ideas and techniques for many centuries. This process was to continue, but whereas in the late medieval period the flow of ideas and technologies was mainly *into* Europe, the period after 1500 saw the flow beginning to reverse. The growing economic

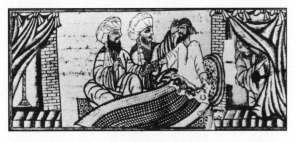

Figure 2.12 A medical consultation in Hamadan, shortly before the death in 1151 of the Shah, Mesnt bin Mehmed bin Melik.

strength of Europe, the importation, mainly from China, of such things as horse harnesses, looms, paper, gunpowder ('Chinese snow') and the magnetic compass, were the foundations of world conquest. By the late fifteenth century the voyages of discovery — by Columbus, Vasco da Gama, and Magellan — had reached round the globe, and East and West Indies had both been seized. Later in the book we will again take up the development of health care elsewhere in the world. You will then see that many of the changes in British and European health care after 1500 that are examined in the following chapters were not confined to Britain or Europe — they too were to change the rest of the world.

Objectives for Chapter 2

When you have studied this chapter you should be able to:

2.1 Explain why modern health care is regarded as having originated in ancient Greece. Factors include the emergence of a naturalistic approach; the development of medical practice as a distinct occupation encompassing treatment, prevention and caring; the emergence of medical schools and the establishment of rules of conduct for physicians.

2.2 Describe how Roman health care differed from that of the Greeks, and show how such differences reflected differences in the political and social structures of the two societies.

2.3 Explain how the Christian church came to dominate health care in western Europe; the way it differed from that of the Graeco-Roman era; and its lasting impact on European health care.

2.4 List the ways in which new secular powers began to replace those of the Church in the running of health care institutions and the administration of public health measures, and the reasons for this.

2.5 Describe how early European health care was influenced by other systems in India, China and the Islamic world.

Questions for Chapter 2

1 (*Objective 2.1*) Even when Hippocratic medicine became established in ancient Greece many people continued to seek cures for their illnesses by worshipping the god of healing, Aesculapius. (The historian of medicine, Henry Sigerist, has cited the Roman Catholic shrine at Lourdes as the nearest modern-day parallel to the Aesculapian approach.) In what ways did Hippocratic medicine differ from the Aesculapian pattern of care?

2 (*Objective 2.2*) 'If the Greeks pointed the way in public health measures, it was the Romans who fully developed this approach.' In what ways is this true, and why might this be so?

3 (*Objective 2.3*)
The Christians of Rome were possessed of a very considerable wealth ... many among their proselytes had sold their lands and houses to increase the public riches of the sect, at the expense indeed of their unfortunate children, who found themselves beggars because their parents had been saints. (Cited in Goody, 1983, p.98)

This somewhat acerbic view of the Christian church was held by Edward Gibbon, the great eighteenth-century historian of the later Roman Empire and what he termed 'the sect'. What point was he making?

4 (*Objective 2.4*)
It does not appear that any sanitary regulations existed from the seventh to the fourteenth centuries. In those dark ages people lived without rule of any kind and consequently frightful epidemics often appeared to desolate the land. (Lemuel Shattuck 1850, quoted in Brockington, 1975, p.86)

Do you agree with Shattuck's view of public health in the late medieval period?

5 (*Objective 2.5*) How important a part did the Islamic world play in the development of European health care?

3

Transitions: the early modern period in British health care

In his description of society in late medieval Europe, the modern French historian Fernand Braudel has laid particular emphasis on *diversity* — the Church and the towns, the landlords and the emerging nation-states were all competing for power and influence:

> This was not one society then but several, coexisting, resting on each other to greater or lesser degree; not one system but several; not one hierarchy but several; not one order but several ... We must think of everything in the plural. (Braudel, 1982, pp.464–5)

☐ In Braudel's terms, which 'societies' had dominated health care during the medieval period?

■ The Church had dominated the early medieval period, while the towns had gained increasing control during the later period.

The struggle between different 'societies' for control continued throughout the early modern period of European history (1500–1800), culminating in the French and Industrial Revolutions of the late eighteenth century, and the eventual dominance of the nation-state.

But although the fully-developed nation-state of the nineteenth century was to be a product of north-western Europe, its origins lay in northern Italy in the thirteenth century.

Independent cities, such as Venice, Pisa and Genoa had expanded rapidly on the basis of Mediterranean trade and developed a large and powerful merchant class. Important changes had taken place in health care and in those ever more prosperous city-states. It was in those that the first attempts to impose external rules of conduct on physicians was made, with the introduction of licensing. In turn, the

physicians had formed themselves into a powerful guild and thus established a monopoly. The merchant rulers of those city-states had increasingly taken on responsibility for the health of the citizens. Doctors had been employed to care for the poor: for example, by 1324, Venice with a population of about 100 000 had no less than thirteen physicians and eighteen surgeons paid for by the city. In addition, fear of the repeated epidemics that swept through Europe had led these city-states to set up health councils and public health boards to seek ways of preventing outbreaks. Nothing like this was being attempted in the rest of Europe at that time, and Italians visiting England commented regularly on the laxity of English public health provisions. By the sixteenth century, however, England had also begun to experience these changes.

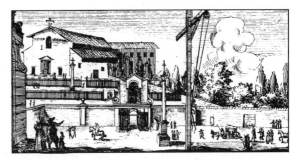

Figure 3.1 The Lazaretto of St Pancrazia in Rome, during the plague epidemic of 1656–1657. The pulley in the foreground was used to inflict punishment on anyone violating the orders of the Health Officers, officials employed by the city to enforce regulations intended to prevent outbreaks.

Religious upheaval: the sixteenth century

At the beginning of the sixteenth century there were four main aspects to health care in Britain. First, there was a plethora of formal practitioners including university-trained physicians, bone-setters, midwives, barber-surgeons and many more. Second, there were public health measures enforced by the towns and cities. Third, there was some assistance and welfare for the poor and destitute, provided by the church, charity and the towns. Fourth, as always, there was surely a vast amount of lay care, although little is known of it.

The power of the Church had been declining throughout the late medieval period. By the sixteenth century, monarchs of newly powerful nation-states viewed the Church's lands and prerogatives with some irritation; merchants in the major towns and cities wondered how the Church's wealth might be put to some more *profitable* use; and a great mass of people viewed the Church as decadent and corrupt. In his *Supplicacyon for the Beggers*, written in 1529, Simon Fish argued:

> But whate remedye to releve us yoore sike, lame and sore bedmen? To make many hospitals for the relief of the poore people? Nay surely. The moo the worse, for ever the fatte of the hole foundation hangeth on the prestes berdes [beards]. (Cited in Rosen, 1963, p.15)

As the power of the Church declined, secular power rose. The state, for example, introduced regulations in three main areas: the licensing of formal practitioners, the stipulation of public health measures, and the establishment of the Poor Laws (of which more shortly). In 1512 it passed 'An Acte concernyage the approbation of physicyons and surgeons'. The preamble declared that:

> ... the science and cunning of physic and surgery ... is daily within this realm exercised by a great multitude of ignorant persons ... [who] boldly and accustomably take upon themselves great cures, and things of great difficulty ... and grievous hurt, damage and destruction of many of the king's liege people. (3 Henry VIII, c.11)

The Act proposed that healers be officially licensed, either by a university or by the local bishop, and that practitioners without that legal permit be subject to substantial fines.

Indeed, this Act of 1512 was only the first of many legal moves in England in the sixteenth century to try to create more coherent healing occupations, bound together by unified systems of licensing and discipline. First, there were the *physicians*, mostly university-educated men. Thomas Linacre, who in 1517 had published a translation of Galen and dedicated it to Henry VIII, obtained a charter from the King in 1518 to establish a College of Physicians of London.

The charter gave the College the power to examine and license physicians, to control practice within seven miles of London, and to monitor the purity of drugs.

Besides the physicians there were, second, the *barber-surgeons*, drawing recruits not through universities but rather through an apprenticeship system similar to other crafts and trades in the towns of the time. In 1540 the surgeons and the more numerous barbers agreed to a charter that brought them together in a United Company. This exempted surgeons from acting as barbers and restricted the surgical operations of barbers to the practice of dentistry. The Company was authorised to fine unlicensed surgeons, although, again, only in the London area.

Third, there were the *apothecaries*, who had evolved as a specialised branch of the grocery trade, maintaining drugs, herbs, balms and spices in their stores or repositories ('*apotheca*' is Latin for a repository). Conflict was intense in the sixteenth century between apothecaries and physicians, for apothecaries could be approached directly by the public for remedies, *without* the mediation of a physician.

The contest between apothecaries and physicians in sixteenth-century England was a forerunner of an issue that is still very much alive today: the degree to which doctors should control medicines through prescription.

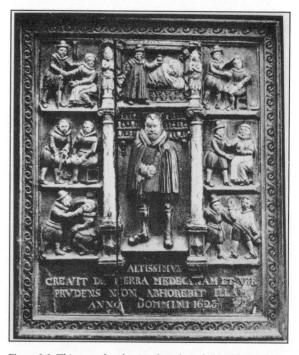

Figure 3.2 This carved and painted signboard, dated 1623, shows the various services available from the Dorset apothecary who displayed it.

And, finally, there were the *midwives*. Midwives were not mentioned in the 1512 Act, but were licensed under its provisions soon afterwards. However, unlike the physicians, surgeons and apothecaries, they were made responsible solely to the bishops.

☐ Considering the nature of midwives' work, can you suggest any reason why this should have been so?
■ Midwifery was concerned with a number of issues in which the Church had, and still has, a keen interest. These included the prevention of abortion, the establishment of paternity, ensuring that unmarried women did not abandon their children, and making sure that births took place in a sound religious atmosphere.

Although each type of practitioner had a distinct role, in practice some of them overlapped considerably. Some midwives, for example, clearly practised general medicine, and some surgeons strayed into the territory of the physicians.

In the early days of medicine at Salerno, physicians and surgeons had stood on an equal basis, but over the centuries the former had become the province of gentlemen educated in classical culture at the universities, while surgery, in England at least, was essentially a *craft* learned by apprenticeship. As Margaret Pelling, a medical historian, has pointed out, the barber-surgeons ran a kind of grooming service for men-about-town:

There seem to have been few limits to the personal services offered by barber-surgeons. Among these, bloodletting and toothdrawing are well known; but barber-surgeons also cleaned teeth by scraping them, pared nails, picked or syringed ears … Barber-surgeons' shops in towns and cities emerge as places of resort for men, offering music, drink, gaming, conversation and news, as well as the services already mentioned. After 1600 many added to their attractions by selling tobacco, a contemporary obsession which first earned credit for curing diseases, including venereal disease. Direct evidence is hard to find, but it seems plausible to propose that the barbershop also served as the first port of call for advice on sexual matters, being, unlike the brothel itself, primarily a male preserve. (Many were located in or next to the red light districts — the 'stews'.) (Pelling, 1985b, forthcoming, pp.19–20)

Besides licensing and controlling the various roles in health care, the state intervened by introducing regulations to reduce environmental hazards to health. For example, in 1532 an Act of Parliament provided for the institution of Commissioners of Sewers in all parts of the kingdom to be responsible for the inspection, construction, amendment and removal of any impediments to rivers.

However, most responsibility for public health remained a local affair. For example, during a plague epidemic in London in 1583 the Privy Council pressed the mayor and aldermen of the city to:

see that all infected houses were shut up and provisions made to feed and maintain the sick persons therein and for preventing their going abroad; that all infected houses were marked; the streets thoroughly cleansed … (Simon, 1890, p.95)

☐ Public health measures, such as those described, had only a limited effect in preventing disease. Can you suggest any reasons why this was so?
■ The measures themselves were inappropriate for stopping the spread of plague,* and the regulations were frequently not enforced.

In practice, effective power remained at a local level, either in the hands of secular or religious authorities. For instance, outside London, there was no College of Physicians to enforce the licensing system: this was instead left to bishops who, given the religious upheavals of the sixteenth century, were occupied elsewhere for much of the time. In the Norwich diocese, for example, ecclesiastical medical licensing only began in earnest in 1583 and midwives were not systematically licensed until the 1630s — yet Norwich was the second city after London. Moreover, even in London the College had a hard time trying to enforce its rule.

The attempts of the state to distinguish between and license different types of practitioner had little immediate effect on the regulation of health care work. A surprisingly large number of practitioners, possibly as many as one for every 200–400 of the population, continued to provide a wide range of services. Few of these people were full-time practitioners: surgeons were, in addition, likely to be craftsmen or work in agriculture.

Health care and the poor
Health care was provided on what would nowadays be called a *'two-tier' system*. The better-off paid privately for whatever services they needed while the poor depended on a mixture of private charity and public funds. Partly because of this we know far more about the care of the poor than we do about that of other classes of society. The institutions that catered for the poor — the hospitals, almshouses and parishes — were all official bodies that kept systematic written records for the inspection of municipal or ecclesiastical authorities. Many of these

*Plague is discussed in greater detail in *Medical Knowledge: Doubt and Certainty, ibid.* (U205 Book II).

records still survive and therefore enable some kind of estimate of the nature and quality of the service.

In the sixteenth century the poor formed a significant proportion of European society. A census of the poor conducted in Norwich in 1570 found that they constituted a quarter of the resident population, half of the poor were also described as sick, disabled or aged. Poverty was an increasing problem at this time partly as a result of rapid population growth and agricultural changes uprooting the traditional peasantry. The towns and cities thus found themselves with the primary responsibility for providing health care and relief for an increasing number of poor people driven off the land. This problem produced a debate about social assistance that is still continuing today, concerning attitudes towards poverty.

Legislation in 1531 in England for poor relief took the view that, apart from the sick and infirm, who were seen as deserving of help, the rest of the poor had only themselves to blame, as being undeserving of assistance. A distinction was therefore drawn between 'aged, poor and impotent persons' who could not work and should therefore be licensed to beg, and 'persons being whole and mighty in body and able to labour'. These were to be 'tied to the end of a cart naked and . . . beaten with whips throughout the same market town or place until his body be bloody'.

Such legislation proved difficult to implement, and in 1536 another attempt suggested a very different approach. It ordered every parish to 'succour, find and keep all and every of the same poor people by way of voluntary and charitable alms . . . in such wise as none of them of necessity shall be compelled to wander idly and go openly in begging'. This legislation was strengthened first in 1552 with the appointment of two commissioners in every parish to go round and collect donations (with the power to fine those who did not contribute), and again in 1576, when 'houses of correction' for 'rogues and idlers' who would not work were set up. These institutions were modelled on one which had been established by the corporation of London in 1555 at the old royal palace near St Bride's Well. They thus became known as 'Bridewells'.

Thus, the sixteenth-century English held a variety of attitudes to poor relief. This had a major bearing on developments in health care because the provision of health care for the poor was closely tied to other forms of poor relief. As there was never at any stage a national system of health care, what was done in one locality often varied radically in other parts of the country: the story must be pieced together from fragments.

Throughout the country, the charitable religious hospitals of the medieval period were being taken over by town councils. In addition, some towns employed doctors to care for the 'deserving' poor. The scale of the task facing some towns was immense: for example, late in the sixteenth century, Norwich with a total population of about 10 000 had 2 000 beggars in the town. Many of them were official, the council having granted licences to those who had a worthy cause for which to beg. In 1570, no less than 200 licences were issued. The council themselves directly hired medical practitioners to treat the sick poor, but unlike the continental methods of appointing salaried town doctors, which had been adopted by a few towns in Britain, Norwich chose to rely principally on hiring practitioners separately for each case. The contracts they issued were usually conditional: the practitioner was paid something on account and a balance if a cure was effected. Only in a few exceptional cases, such as the skilled bone-setter Richard Durrant, did the council eventually pay a regular salary.

☐ To what extent do you think the provision of health care and assistance was an appropriate response to the needs of the poor?

■ While such help would have provided some immediate relief of suffering, it would have made no contribution to preventing poverty.

Improvements in public health measures were also a matter for local action. Recognition of the need for improvements is apparent from civic records. For example, records for London make frequent reference to the need for cleansing and conservation of ditches in the city, of the need for pavements to be built and maintained and for filth to be removed. Similarly the problems of overbuilding and overcrowding are constantly mentioned. Local improvements, such as a town water supply, were paid for either by wealthy benefactors or by local taxes. In 1585, for instance, an Act of Parliament provided for the construction of the Plymouth Water leat devised by Sir Francis Drake, then a member of the town council. The leat brought water by means of gravity from Dartmouth about 24 miles away. Compared with the genius of the Romans, however, water supplies to many towns remained rudimentary for much of the sixteenth century. In London, for example, in 1599 Thomas Platter, a 'Traveller', described how:

Spring or drinking water . . . enclosed in great, well sealed stone cisterns in different parts of the town is let off through cocks into special wooden iron-bound vessels with broad bottoms and narrow tops, which poor labourers carry to and fro to the house on their shoulders and sell.

Public lavatories in this period also never reached the luxury established by the Romans. There do, however, seem to have been quite a large number of them in Elizabethan London, particularly at the riverside end of narrow lanes. In wealthier homes the smelly 'garderobes' or privys were also being replaced by 'stoolhouses' each with its 'close-stool' — a sort of commode — and some had elaborate drainage systems. For example, in Ingateston Hall in Essex, Sir William Petre built five stoolhouses and 'divers vaults and gutters of brick, very large under the ground round about the whole situation of the house, conveying waters from every office'. But, of course, no system of sewers existed to which such 'waters' could be conveyed: they were simply moved away from the immediate vicinity of the Hall.

The seventeenth century: the perspective of the state

The Italian city-states had for many centuries led the way in both commerce and medicine, but during the seventeenth century Holland and England came increasingly to dominate both. Through a massive expansion in world trade England became, by 1700, the wealthiest country in Europe, and London, with 900 000 people, by far the largest city. The change came rapidly. England, a medical backwater in the early seventeenth century, developed its own major scientific tradition in medicine in the hands of such people as William Harvey and Thomas Sydenham. The English Revolution, which dominated the middle decades of the century, was associated with a fundamental rethinking of many social and political issues. This affected health care in three important ways: (a) the expansion of *scientific work* in medicine, evidenced by the dramatic rise in medical book production after 1650 (Figure 3.3) and the start of clinical teaching, including human dissection; (b) further attempts to enforce *state regulations* and control on locally based authority, though with only limited success; and (c) the emergence of the concept of statistical evidence and a greater awareness of the concept of *population*.

Prior to the emergence of the territorial nation-state, the concept of population was not well established. Why was this the case? One answer seems to be that it was only after the nation-state had appeared that there was a constant need to define the people within its borders, and to 'count heads'. This concern with counting resulted in the creation of *statistics*, a word of German origin whose root is '*der Staat*': the state. In 1603, during one of London's worst plagues, the City of London had begun to record systematically weekly statistics on christenings and burials. In 1662 John Graunt became the first person to demonstrate the use of statistics as a powerful method of social analysis. His publication, entitled *Natural and Political Observations made upon the Bills of Mortality*, was based on these statistics. For the first time, population statistics were used as data from which to draw inferences and make hypotheses. As the British philosopher, Ian Hacking, observes, there was:

> ... no holding back Graunt's inventive mind. The course of various diseases across the decades, the number of inhabitants, the ratio of females to males, the proportion of people dying at several ages, the number of men fit to bear arms, the emigration from city to country in times of fever, the influence of the plague upon birth rates, and the projected growth of London: all these subjects are examined with gusto. (Hacking, 1984, p.106)

The importance of Graunt's work was recognised almost immediately. To take one example which was to have an extraordinary impact: once the concept of life expectancy at different ages and for different sexes and classes of population had been established from his mortality tables, the business of *insurance* against death or ill-health became much more practicable; indeed, insurance has become one of the most important methods of funding health care in the twentieth century. Graunt, therefore, was representative of an exceedingly powerful system of thought, and the Royal Society, considering his admission, was told in forthright terms by Charles II that 'if they found any more such tradesmen they should be sure to admit them without any more ado'.

Medical thought and practice

The development of statistics in England was accompanied by the shift of the centre of medical thought from Italy to northern Europe. As regards the teaching of medicine, it was the Dutch, rather than the English, who took the dominant position from the Italians. By the late sixteenth century, medical teaching had been introduced to the University of Leyden and from 1626 this included bedside teaching, a central component of the new scientific approach. Leyden became an international centre of medical education for, amongst others, British physicians, for at that time there was no clinical teaching along Italian lines in England, nor was there dissection.

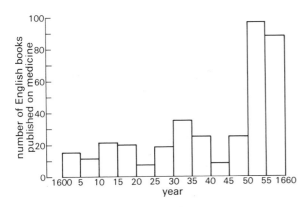

Figure 3.3 The number of English books on medicine published in five-yearly periods from 1600 to 1660.
(Source: data derived from Webster, 1975, Figure 2, p.489)

Table 3.1 Physicians and population in selected European towns 1575 to 1675

| Town | Year | Number of physicians | | Total | Population (000s) | Ratio (per 10 000) |
		Within College	Outside College			
Florence	1630	12	21	33	80	4.1
Pisa	1630			12	13	9.2
Palermo	1575			22	80	2.7
Milan	1591	37	not known	not known	100	>3.7
Bologna	1630			>42	62	>6.8
Rome	1675	14	150	164	130	12.6
Antwerp	1585			18	80	2.2
Rouen	1605	16		16	80	2.0
Lyons	1620	20		20	90	2.2
Paris	1626			85	300	2.1
Amsterdam	1641			50	135	3.7

(Source: derived from Cipolla, 1976b, Table 2, p.82)

Training abroad, however, was expensive, and there were very few academically trained doctors in Britain. Between 1620 and 1640 the University of Oxford produced an annual average of only two and a half MBs (Bachelor of Medicine) and one MD (Doctor of Medicine). Cambridge, the only other university in England, did even worse, averaging one and one and a half respectively. The situation in other areas of western Europe was very different, as Table 3.1 shows.

□ What does it tell you about the supply of physicians in different parts of continental Europe?

■ That there was at least a six-fold difference between different cities. Rome, for example had more than twelve physicians for every ten thousand of its inhabitants, compared with about two per ten thousand in French towns.

The situation in northern Italy was even more remarkable than these figures indicate, for not only were there large numbers of university-trained doctors in the cities, but there were many of them in the rural areas as well. Tuscany in 1630 had a rural population of about 550 000 served by at least fifty-five trained physicians, an extraordinarily high prevalence for a rural area of a pre-industrial society.

□ What is the main limitation of the data in Table 3.1 for assessing the provision of medical care in the seventeenth century?

■ Table 3.1 includes information on trained physicians only, who were but one of a number of different occupations providing care.

Finally, in addition to all these various sorts of practitioner there were many religious and magical cures and a whole host of people offering secret remedies for a price.

Unlicensed practitioners were referred to as 'quacks', a delightful word still in use: it is probably an abbreviation of 'quack salver' which itself derives from the Dutch 'kwakken', to prattle, and 'salf', to salve or heal. It was originally used by physicians to describe anyone boasting their skills from the pulpit, lectern or market-place. In the eyes of the licensed practitioners, quacks were phony doctors who set out to deceive the public with bogus and useless remedies.

□ Do you think that the physicians' critical attitude was tenable?

■ It wasn't. Quacks' remedies were probably no more or less ineffective than those of the physicians.

Few people could afford to consult a physician and depended instead on unlicensed practitioners. In addition, if people wanted specialist care, they were obliged to turn to the quacks, for while college physicians, like their Greek predecessors, were generalists, trained in a common body of knowledge, quacks and mountebanks often specialised, for example, in bone-setting, eye disease or kidney stones; so, too, did women.

Although excluded from university training and thus from being physicians, women made up a fairly high proportion of the overall number of practitioners. The medical historians, Margaret Pelling and Charles Webster, have estimated that at the end of the sixteenth century women may have constituted about a quarter of all the practitioners in London and one third of the healers hired by the council in Norwich to treat the sick poor (Pelling, 1985b, forthcoming; Pelling and Webster, 1979).

Women played three other important roles as formal carers. One was nursing of various kinds. Apart from the nurses to be found in hospitals, parishes regularly

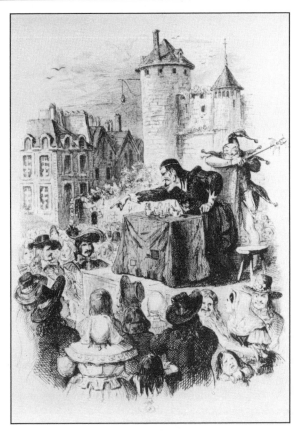

Figure 3.4 A quack or mountebank (from the Italian *monta in banco* — 'mount on bench') at work.

employed women to nurse orphans or to give lodging to the sick poor, while the wet-nurse and the children's nurse were a common part of the establishment of richer families. London babies were commonly sent for wet-nursing to the outlying villages, a practice that continued throughout Britain, France and Germany right up to the present century.

The second role was a forerunner of the nineteenth-century health visitor. Women were employed during plague epidemics as 'discreet persons' to check that infected people were abiding by the public health regulations imposed by the town or city council. In contrast, the third role for women was rather less formal. Right into the nineteenth century a good deal of health care in rural areas was provided free of charge by the local gentry or clergy, or more often, by their wives. This was an ancient tradition, which survives, though somewhat changed, in the voluntary work of today. The following extract is from the diary of Lady Margaret Hoby in 1601:

this day, in the afternone, I had a child brought to me that was born at Silpho, one Talliour sonne, who had no fundament [anus] and had no passage for excrementes but at the Mouth; I was ernestly intreated to Cutt the place to see if any passhage could be made, but, although I Cutt deepe and searched, there was none to be found. (Cited in Wyman, 1984, pp.31–2)

Books were printed to aid lay care. *The Surgion's Directorie* of 1652, for example, was addressed 'to all the Vertuous Ladyes and Gentlewomen of this Common-Wealth of England'.

Books such as this were, in their day, radical publications. The College of Physicians opposed attempts to translate medical works into the vernacular. Indeed, in Charles I's reign (1625–1649) they cooperated willingly with the censorship of medical publications. Nicholas Culpeper, one of whose many works, the *Herbal* is still regularly published, was a major opponent of measures to withhold medical knowledge from lay people. As he stated in the preface to one of his books, he had had a vision in which:

All the sick People in England presented themselves before me, and told me They had Herbes in their Gardens that might cure them, but knew not the vertues of them. (Cited in Webster, 1975, p.271)

☐ Apart from censorship, what factors can you think of that might have limited the spread of health care books at this time?
■ The main factors were the low level of literacy and the high cost of books.

There is no reliable information on how many (or few) people could read or write at this time: the culture was in many respects an oral one. As to the cost of books, it had been falling, but slowly: in the thirteenth century the parchment for one large bible consumed the hides of 200–300 sheep; by the fifteenth century '... the annual salary of an average professor in the University of Pavia, if entirely spent on books, would purchase less than two volumes of law ... and ten in medicine' (White, 1976, pp.160 and 162); by the seventeenth century, costs had fallen to around a quarter of the fifteenth-century level, but not till the nineteenth century were they within reach of a mass market.

Hospitals: a changing climate of ideas
Institutional care did not change greatly in seventeenth-century Britain. The healing of the sick remained only a small part of the traditional notion of a hospital. There were proposals for a model teaching hospital to be created in London, for the establishment of a national salaried

service of doctors and surgeons, and for the creation of hospitals in every county and city where the poor would be treated free of charge. In practice the only developments were the establishment of the clinical teaching of doctors in St Bartholomew's Hospital, and an increasing number of physicians being attached to hospitals (on the grounds that medical attention might not only help some patients, but would prove cheaper in the long run as some inmates' stay would thereby be lessened).

By contrast, in France, fundamental changes in the role of hospitals were underway. *Hôtels-Dieu* were created which catered solely for the sick. They were located particularly in the more prosperous north and were staffed principally by surgeons — physicians normally shunned them. They treated the poor, but excluded certain categories of patient — the mad, the incurable, those suffering from venereal disease or scrofula (tuberculosis), and even, in some cases, women. Besides in-patient care the surgeons also began to run out-patient clinics.

Although there was no equivalent change in the organisation of institutional care in England, the new science of *statistics* was starting to make some impact, in the hands of a contemporary of Graunt's, William Petty. His series of essays on the applications of statistics — *'political arithmetic'*, as he styled the subject — constitutes one of the earliest examples of what we would now call economics. Like Graunt, Petty took as his starting point an analysis of Bills of Mortality, but his analyses took him into a number of new areas. First, he realised that statistics could be used to conduct controlled experiments on the way health care was provided, for example, '... whether of 100 sick of acute diseases who use physicians, as many die in misery as where no art is used, or only chance' (cited in Hacking, 1984, p.105). In a lecture in 1676, he turned his attention to the provision of hospitals:

Another cause of defect in the art of medicine and consequently of its contempt is that there have not been hospitals for the accommodation of sick people ... a man shall learn in a well regulated hospital, where he may within halfe a hower's time observe his choice of 1 000 patients, more in one yeare than in 10 without it, even by reading the best books that can be written. (Cited in Woodward, 1974, p.7)

□   What changes in the role of the hospital was Petty advocating?

■   He was arguing for two main changes: first, that hospitals should specialise in admitting people who were sick, and by implication should not be expected to admit many classes of people who were also using them; second, that hospitals and practical learning rather than books and theoretical learning would be the best way for medical understanding to advance.

In the event, it was to be well over a hundred years before these ideas were fully realised in England. However, Petty was simultaneously opening up other areas of inquiry. In particular, he forged a link between the health of the population and its monetary value to the state. The way he did so now seems crude, but the important thing was not the technique, but rather the thought that the state had vested economic interests in the population's health; and that life had a *value* (around £70 per life, reckoned Petty). The applications were endless: if plague killed 100 000 people, the cost to the nation would be £7 million; by spending £70 000 the state could save more than 100 times as much; if the government were to provide lying-in hospitals for illegitimate children, at a cost of only 30 shillings per child, it would avoid a likely death an obtain a handsome return from a lifetime's labour, and so on.

Poor Laws and public health

Part of the social background to Petty's work lay in the efforts by the state during the seventeenth century to establish a national system of poor relief. You have already seen that the poor were an object of social policy in sixteenth-century England. In 1598, and again in 1601, a variety of regulations and laws were brought together by Parliament, and the Acts of these years are conventionally taken as the beginnings of the *Poor Law*: laws for raising local taxes and appointing officials to act as overseers of the poor. The philosophy behind the Poor Laws changed over time, as you will see, but always contained a mixture of relief for those unable to work, and compulsory activities — for example, in *workhouses* provided under Poor Law regulations — to 'keep idle hands busy'.

The Poor Law system is important in the historical development of health care in Britain, for many of the provisions made for the poor entailed some form of medical provision.

Discussion of Poor Law medical services in this and the next chapter will concentrate on *institutional* care. There are two main reasons for this: first, many of the buildings erected under the Poor Law auspices are still used for health care purposes, and second, it is in the nature of public institutions that records are kept, yielding data for modern research.

But poor relief and medical relief were also provided to people in their homes, and such *outdoor* relief, although alternately encouraged and discouraged, was an ever-present part of the Poor Law system. Data on outdoor relief are fragmentary and it is difficult to state precisely how many people were receiving what kind of services. Outdoor relief is therefore less prominent in the following pages than its importance warrants.

The Poor Law system was to form an important part of

life in Britain for centuries, and did not formally disappear until 1948 with the passing of the National Assistance Act.

The Poor Laws of 1598 and 1601 were important for three reasons: (a) they demonstrated the acceptance of society's responsibility towards the poor and the need to enforce it; (b) they established *in statute* the distinction between the 'deserving' and 'undeserving' poor; and (c) they established local machinery for the maintenance of the poor which became increasingly inseparable from the provision of health care.

The extract from the Preamble to the 1598 Act gives some indication of the reasons behind it:

> Whereas a good part of the strength of this realm consisteth in the number of good and able subjects and of late years more than in time past there have been sundry towns, parishes and houses of husbandry destroyed and become desolate where a great number of poor people are become wanderers, idle and loose, which is the cause of infinite inconvenience. (Cited in Bruce, 1968, p.36)

□ What three factors appear to have motivated the passing of the Act?
■ 1 A concern with the 'strength of this realm' (the Spanish Armada was a recent and vivid event).
2 Feeling and concern about the destruction of villages.
3 Fear of wandering 'vagrants' and the 'inconvenience' they caused.

One of the effects of the Act was that it gradually replaced the tradition of licensed begging. For example:

> Till the breaking out of Civil Warres, Tom O'Bedlams did travel about the countrey. They had been poore distracted men that had been putt into Bedlam where, recovering to some sobernesse, they were licentiated to goe a-begging ... they wore about their necks a great horn of an oxe in a string of bawdric, which, when they came to an house for almes, they did wind, and they did put the drink given to them into their horns, where they did put a stopple. (John Aubrey, cited in Rosen, 1958, p.153)

During the seventeenth century 'pauper lunatics' such as those described by the contemporary writer, John Aubrey, were handled in a variety of different ways. They might be placed in the old leprosaria, or the new Bridewells; placed in the care of an individual who would be paid for this service; or made the responsibility of the entire parish. There was therefore, in theory at least, a fairly extensive system of ways and means by which they might be cared for or controlled. Which option was chosen depended not just on the mental condition of the person but on their relative wealth, for care of the insane remained primarily a family

affair, and those with money were expected to pay for their care or confinement, sometimes through the appointment of individual carers and sometimes through the use of private madhouses: the suburb of Hoxton, in London, became famous for its private madhouses.

The need for some form of official supervision of the care of the insane would have been vital because of the emphasis on physically violent treatment at that time. The following is taken from an early seventeenth-century summary of the *Common Law of England* written for Justices of the Peace:

> it is lawful for the parents, kinsmen, or other friends of a man that is mad, or frantic (who being at liberty attempteth to burn a house or to do some other mischief, or to hurt himself or others) to take him and put him into an house, to bind or chain him, and to beat him with rods, and to do any other forcible act to reclaim him, or to keep him so as he shall do not hurt. (Cited in Alldridge, 1979, pp.324–5)

Responsibility for supervision under the 1598 Act rested with Justices of the Peace, a medieval office, whose powers were vastly expanded by the Tudor state. Though the work of JPs was unpaid, the local gentry willingly undertook office, for the JP had considerable influence and standing in his locality. It would be wrong, however, to imagine that the Poor Laws actually established an effective national system, funded mainly by rates, and making clear distinctions between different types of indigent person. In practice, it has been suggested that in the years up to 1660 voluntary donations still constituted as much as 90 per cent of the total volume of funds intended for poor relief.

The Acts of 1598 and 1601 were just one part of the attempt to develop a uniform national system. Similar attempts were taking place throughout northern Europe. For example, an idea of the extent of such activity in Germany can be gained from the list of 'Regulations of police in the City of Nuremburg' (Table 3.2).

□ What strikes you about the list?
■ Two things may have done: the meaning of the word 'police' has altered significantly; and attempts

Table 3.2 Regulations of police of the City of Nuremburg

Police of security	Police of health and cleanliness
Police of customs	Police of building/manufactures
Police of commerce	Fire regulations
Police of trades	Police of forests and hunting
Police of foodstuffs	Control of beggars
	Police of Jews

(Source: derived from Pasquino, 1978, p.46)

were being made to regulate a very wide range of activities.

Regulations reached into almost every nook and cranny of the social fabric: how a parent should address a child, what should be eaten at wedding-feasts, what animals could cross a bridge, what rights different houses had over water supplies, and so on. One recent bibliography of the subject traced no less than 3 215 publications on the 'science of police' that appeared in German-speaking areas of Europe during the seventeenth and eighteenth centuries alone.

Despite such regulations, virtually no European power could govern effectively at the local level. Ancient local powers were too great and communications were lacking, as was an efficient and uncorrupt administrative apparatus. For example, a plague epidemic in 1663–1665 prompted the first English quarantine on a national scale. In 1663, in response to the knowledge that plague had broken out in many other countries, the Mayor and Aldermen of London advised the King that, after the custom of other countries, vessels coming from infected ports should not initially be permitted to come nearer than Gravesend. In addition, no ship was allowed to enter the Port of London without a Bill of Health from the authorities of the port from which they had sailed. However, the ease with which such bills could be forged is illustrated in the following extract from the diary of a ship's surgeon written in the middle of the seventeenth century concerning his ship's entrance to the port of Genoa:

> When we came in our merchants came by us but durst not come on board ... we had no bill of health to certify the place not having the pest whence we came. Wherefore I set my wits and drew up one as from Governor of Newfoundland and signed myself as Secretary ... This passed for current and ... admitted, we lay there ... (Cited in Harrison and Royston, 1963, pp.259–60)

For the most part, public health measures remained subject to local initiatives (or local inertia) throughout the seventeenth century. The major problems remained those of sanitation and water supply: 'Every street', wrote a traveller to Edinburgh in 1705,

> shows the nastiness of the inhabitants: the excrements lie in heaps. In a morning the scent was so offensive that we were forc'd to hold our noses as we past streets and take care where we trod for fear of disobliging our shoes, and to walk in the middle at night for fear of an accident to our heads. (Cited in Doyle, 1978, p.128)

Edinburgh was notorious in such matters. How far it was typical is hard to say. It was certainly claimed that Berlin could be smelt from a mile away and better-off people left London in summer to avoid the stench of the River Thames. Probably most western European towns and cities of this period were relatively similar.

Although there was little improvement in sanitation, there were some developments in water supplies, through the activities of parishes (the 'parish pump') and also by private action. In 1609, Sir Hugh Middleton privately financed the construction of a channel to bring water to London from springs in Middlesex and Hertfordshire. The New River Company was a technical success, but a financial flop, and the use of private business enterprise to try to carry out public functions developed slowly. In the diary of Celia Fiennes, who travelled extensively from 1685 to 1698, Leicester is so described:

> they have a water house and a water mill to turn the water into the pipes to serve the town, as it is in London it comes but once a day so they save the water in deep leaden tubbs ... there are wells in some streets to draw water by a hand wheele for the common use of the town. (Cited in Harrison and Royston, 1963, p.15)

By the late seventeenth century, however, the combination of private and parish enterprise and a series of important technical developments was slowly producing improvements in water supplies. An Italian, L.A. Porzio, had developed the idea of using sand to filter water, and in France filters for household use were introduced. And in Germany, with its long tradition of mining technology, pumps began to be used for the supply of water in towns. As with other developments in health care in the seventeenth century, the full benefits were not to be felt until later. In many ways the seventeenth century was a period of consolidation and preparation. Fundamental intellectual changes took place, such as the development of the 'population' perspective, but little in the way of practical improvements to health.

The emergence of modern health care: the eighteenth century

The eighteenth century in northern Europe was a period of accelerating social change. Increasingly people moved from the countryside to the new urban centres of industry and trade. In Britain, whereas before 1700 London had been the only city of any size, in the eighteenth century, new cities began to spring up: the population of Bristol rose from 20 000 to 64 000; Glasgow from 13 000 to 84 000; and, most spectacular of all, Manchester, which, in less than 25 years, trebled its population to reach 84 000 by 1801. By this last date one quarter of the population of England was living in urbanised south Lancashire.

During the seventeenth century, population growth and

changes in land ownership had led to an increase in landless peasants. These trends, affecting much of Europe, continued, and by the end of the eighteenth century over 30 per cent of the French rural population may have been reduced to beggary. Many headed for the towns. In Paris it is estimated at this time that one quarter of the population was unemployed, in Lyons, one sixth and in London, one-eighth. A graphic illustration of the extent of urban poverty is the number of abandoned children. In 1772 in Paris, which was particularly affected, 7 676 foundlings were taken into care — no less than 40 per cent of all the children baptised in that year in the city.

It was against this background of social upheaval that the intellectual developments of the previous century began to bear fruit in the field of health care. The eighteenth century saw the emergence of modern scientific medicine; not only did natural science research produce some of the first effective treatments, such as the use of citrus fruits for scurvy, but also the role of hospitals was altered to focus their attention on the care of the sick.

Edinburgh and the art of physic

While industrialisation in England, and later in Scotland, led to the creation of appalling urban living conditions for the mass of the population, it also produced enormous national wealth. This in turn led to an increased demand for university-trained doctors to provide private care for the much enlarged middle class and to staff the new hospitals that were being built throughout Britain. There was also an additional demand for doctors on slaving ships, in the expanding number of colonies, and in the military.

□ Where in northern Europe had medical training been expanding in the seventeenth century?
■ The University of Leyden (see page 27).

Leyden's importance was further increased by the appointment to the Chair of Botany and Medicine in 1709 of Hermann Boerhaave, who established the modern system of clinical teaching. Students from all over Europe and even the Americas flocked to his lectures which were given in Latin, still the international language of Europe. Table 3.3 shows the numbers of English-speaking students studying under Boerhaave between 1709 and 1738.

□ What strikes you about the relative numbers from the three countries of the British Isles?
■ The number of Scots was higher than would have been expected considering the size of the Scottish population.

The large number of Scottish students returning home was just one of the factors that led to Edinburgh taking over from Leyden as the international centre of medical thought and training in the second half of the eighteenth century.

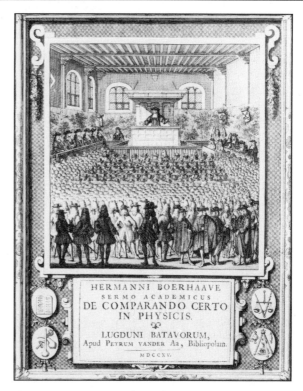

Figure 3.5 Hermann Boerhaave lecturing. Engraving from a publication by P. van der Aa, 1715.

Table 3.3 Origin of English-speaking students of Boerhaave at Leyden, 1709–1738

	Size of population (in 1701, in millions)	Number of students
Angli [English]	5.8	352
Scoti [Scottish]	1.0	244
Hiberni [Irish]	2.5	122
Others	—	28
Total	—	746

(Source: derived from Underwood, 1977, p.24 and Deane and Cole, 1978, p.6)

There were at least three other reasons. First, the surgeons and apothecaries in Scotland had agreed to merge as early as 1657, thus creating an occupation with both surgical and medical skills whose practitioners could claim to be an early form of generalist. Second, the College of Physicians in Edinburgh had not been established until 1681 and as it had much less power than its English counterpart it could not block new developments. And third, Edinburgh had ceased to be an independent political capital after the Union

Table 3.4 Place of training of graduate British medical practitioners, 1600–1850

	Total number	Oxford/ Cambridge (%)	Europe (%)	Scotland (%)
1600–1650	635	94	6	0
1650–1700	1168	80	17	3
1700–1750	1408	44	27	29
1750–1800	3034	8	6	86
1800–1850	8291	3	<1	96

(Source: based on Newman, 1957, p.49)

with England in 1707. The Town Council was determined to use its close ties with the University to create a new role for the city as an international centre of learning — the 'Athens of the North', as it was termed. With Boerhaave's death in 1738, Edinburgh rapidly took action, expanding its new Royal Infirmary to contain 228 beds. Table 3.4 illustrates strikingly the degree to which the centre of gravity in British medical training swung to Scotland.

☐ Apart from the huge growth in Scottish medicine, what trends are revealed in this table about where British doctors trained and about the development of the profession?

■ First, the actual proportion who trained abroad was very small until the period from 1650 to 1750, when it grew and then rapidly declined. Second, more than thirteen times as many doctors were being trained in the final 50 years as in the first. (The population of Britain had grown about fourfold over this same period.)

It should however be remembered that despite the huge increase in training, physicians continued to make up only a small proportion of the total number of formal practitioners in the eighteenth century. For example, an inquiry in Lincolnshire revealed five physicians, with licences from Edinburgh; eleven surgeons and apothecaries supposedly trained by apprenticeship (only one of whom had actually served an apprenticeship but all of whom acted as doctors); 63 midwives; and 40 other healers. Rivalry between the various categories continued, such as the apothecaries' struggle to preserve their right to prescribe as well as dispense medicines. (This issue has re-emerged in a modified form in recent years with demands by pharmacists that they should have the right to question and even substitute alternative medicines equivalent to those which a doctor has prescribed.) Rivalry also existed between the Scottish medical graduates and the English College of Physicians, which refused to recognise the 'Scotch' degrees.

The massive increase in the number of university-trained doctors meant that they, rather than other occupations, began to be employed to provide health care. The Poor Law required that the parishes provided necessary relief for the 'deserving poor'. The church-wardens and four of the wealthier householders were to oversee poor relief, meeting regularly in the vestry for this purpose. The extent and quality of the care provided is a matter of debate. The eighteenth-century poet George Crabbe, who had himself been a doctor, wrote as follows of a medical visit to the poorhouse:

A potent quack, long versed in human ills,
Who first insults the victims whom he kills;
Whose murd'rous hand a drowsy bench protect,
And whose most tender mercy is neglect.
Paid by the parish for attendance here,
He wears contempt upon his sapient sneer
(From *The Village*; cited in Turner, 1958, p.102)

In contrast, E.G. Thomas, a medical historian, has argued that there is considerable evidence in parish records of quite an elaborate system run with some humanity and care. On his account, ordinary cases would often be dealt with by a local 'nurse' or bone-setter and more serious cases by a university-trained doctor:

The humanity of the local doctor could make itself felt too. At Brayton in Berkshire in 1816 the doctor's bill was £20 for a half year. However, 'through the Philanthropy and Disposition of Mr Hayward which he is well known to possess he only charged the parish nine pounds'. (Thomas, 1980, p.3)

☐ How would you explain the discrepancy between these two accounts?

■ There are several possibilities. One is that parish records are limited and are, in any case, official accounts — they may conceal as much as they reveal. Another is that Crabbe is an unreliable witness who may exaggerate grossly for the sake of a good story. Yet a third lies in the intensely local character of health and poor relief administration in this period, which gave rise to considerable variations in the quality of care.

Whichever explanation is correct, Thomas provides considerable evidence of a fairly elaborate system, at least in the south of England. Many cases were the subject of individual contracts; such contracts were made with a wide range of practitioners, not just the university-trained, and in complex cases, there was sometimes a conditional element. For example, in 1758 in the small town of Woodstock just north of Oxford, it was decided: 'to give Mrs Southam two guineas and a half for the cure of James Smith's leg; one guinea to be paid immediately and the other guinea and a half so soon as we are fully satisfy'd of ye cure' (Cited in Thomas, 1980, p.2).

The other trend at this time was the development of a salaried rural medical service; rather than contracting with a range of practitioners for individual cases, parishes began to hire doctors for an annual fee, though this might still be done on a competitive basis with different doctors putting in bids for the business.

While care for the poor remained a local responsibility in England, attempts were made to introduce a more centralised system in France. In 1693 a system was started whereby medicines — *les remédes du Roi* — were sent to

bishops, hospital administrators, lords of the manor, a religious nursing order, and above all, to the rural clergy for free distribution. The scale of all this was small — an order of 1 March 1769 fixed the number of such medicine chests at 742 small chests and 32 large ones. Nevertheless, this measure is an indication of the continued involvement of the clergy in medical care.

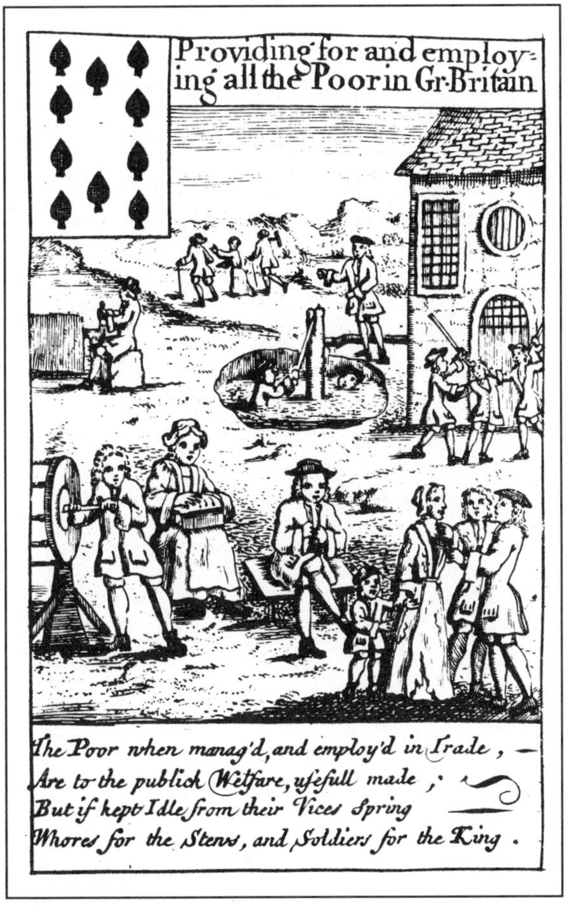

Hospitals: something old, something new

As you have seen, large areas of Britain were rapidly becoming urbanised during the eighteenth century. Along with the growth in the number of university-trained doctors, this led to an important change in the health care of the period — the creation in many of the large towns of new hospitals which catered specifically for the sick.

☐ Was the development of hospitals specifically for the sick a new idea?

■ No. As you have seen, in the seventeenth century the French had developed *Hôtels-Dieu* (see page 30).

The hospitals were essentially private, charitable enterprises catering almost exclusively for the sick poor. The first of these *voluntary hospitals* was the Westminster, founded in London in 1719 by a charitable society led by a banker, 'good Henry' Hoare. The charity took a new form, in part modelled on the 'joint-stock' companies listed on a rapidly expanding stock exchange. It was dependent on voluntary subscriptions or contributions rather than endowments; subscribers rather than governors took care of the administration; and physicians and surgeons held honorary positions, receiving no salary, but having the rights of subscribers, their income being derived from private practice outside the hospitals. At first, parishes sent patients there on an individual basis, but by the early nineteenth century many parishes had linked together and joined a common scheme to send patients to their local hospital. By 1830 at least eighty Oxfordshire parishes — thirty per cent — were paying sums up to six guineas a year to the Radcliffe Infirmary in Oxford as part of such a scheme.

The movement spread rapidly around the country: Edinburgh opened its Royal Infirmary in 1729; St George's in London was created in 1733; Winchester built such a hospital in 1736, followed in quick succession by Bristol (1737), York (1740), Exeter (1741) and Liverpool (1745). By 1780, there were 38 such hospitals in the provinces and by the end of the century most of the cities and larger towns in Britain had their own. As part of this same process, and run in much the same fashion (though with the addition of a Ladies Committee), lying-in or maternity hospitals were created. The first of these was founded in Dublin in 1745 and over the next twenty years no fewer than four of these institutions were created in London. Finally, the British

Figure 3.6 A poorhouse depicted on a playing card of 1720.

colonies in America were quick to imitate the new idea of the voluntary hospital, the first, opening in Philadelphia in 1751, modelled on Edinburgh's.

Though the voluntary hospital was a new form it embodied old ideas. In medieval times hospitals had often raised funds through 'proctors' who wandered the country collecting alms. Now, with a growing urban middle class, charity took new forms: concerts (which supposedly funded most of the Birmingham hospital), balls, and the like, as well as the traditional support from charitable local businessmen or those who wished to look after the health of their workforce; all contributed.

Just like the Poor Law, however, the eighteenth-century voluntary hospital was and is the subject of impassioned debate. There have been three main controversies. First, did it actually cure people, as the managers liked to claim, or was it instead a breeding ground for disease? Opinion has swung back and forth, though a detailed study by John Woodward, a historian, (1974) suggests that things may not have been too bad after all. Second, were they noble monuments to Christian charity or did they instead serve a darker purpose? Charles Webster, for example, has recently described them as:

> an object of civic pride, a conspicuous symbol of the charitable impulses of the rich, and a spur to the gratitude and submission of the poor. (Webster, 1978, p.214)

And, third, for all the spread of the voluntary hospital across Britain during the eighteenth century, did it in fact serve the real medical needs of the poor? Even if Woodward is correct in arguing that conditions were not too insanitary, did the hospitals admit the right people and in sufficient numbers? Webster argues that hospitals built in areas of rapid population growth were quickly swamped. Moreover, although they were new foundations and differed from the traditional hospital in focusing more upon the sick, most operated with a medical remit that had hardly changed. Children, consumptives, epileptics, the dying, the syphilitic, pregnant women and those suffering from infectious disease were still excluded. Above all, perhaps, admission could usually only be obtained through a Letter of Recommendation from a subscriber and after numerous formalities. Eighteenth-century charity had a strongly personal element. Many people enjoyed their powers of patronage and the power to grant or deny entry to the sick poor was a formidable privilege enjoyed by every subscriber.

☐ In what way is this reminiscent of medieval hospitals' charity described in the previous chapter?

■ There, too, there was a strongly personal element. The inmates of medieval hospitals commonly said daily prayers for the soul of the founder and some even wore the livery of their benefactor.

Of rather more importance than the in-patient care provided by voluntary hospitals was another new development, the *dispensary*, a version of the out-patient care started at the *Hotel-Dieu* in Paris in the late seventeenth century. The Royal College of Physicians opened their first dispensary for the poor in 1696, though it closed again in 1725. Nearly fifty years later, Dr George Armstrong tried again, opening the Dispensary for the Infant Poor in Red Lion Square, Holborn, London. The idea caught on rapidly. A Quaker physician opened a further dispensary in 1770 and subsequently fifteen more were opened in London and roughly the same number elsewhere. At the same time, some of the new voluntary

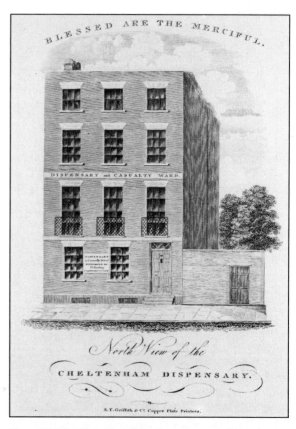

Figure 3.7 The Cheltenham Dispensary, 'supported by voluntary contributions', in 1826. Dispensaries provided services not generally given by the voluntary hospitals: 'Dispensaries are adapted to the cure not only of all chronic and such acute complaints as are uninfectious, but also of epidemic and contagious diseases, when raging (as among the poor is often the case) in the most violent and destructive manner' (Allen, O. (1845) *A History of the York Dispensary*).

Table 3.5 Average new attendances, per year in each decade, at out-patient departments in selected hospitals 1740–1800

Decade	Radcliffe Infirmary Oxford	Gloucester Infirmary	The London Hospital
1740–9			3 756
1750–9		136	7 560
1760–9		154	6 913
1770–9	142	196	
1780–9	247	300	6 830
1790–9	279	391	2 431

(Source: Loudon, 1978, p.974)

hospitals began to open out-patient departments and some even began, eventually, to engage in home visiting. As can be seen in Table 3.5, the numbers attending at Oxford and Gloucester were at first very small, while even the few thousand attendants in London each year must be set alongside a total population approaching one million in the latter part of the century.

Nevertheless, such a service potentially offered the possibility of medical care far cheaper than that of in-patients, though it was still restricted by the need for a Letter of Recommendation. Only a few free dispensaries allowed people to refer themselves for treatment.

Care of the mentally ill and retarded also altered during this period. In addition to the private madhouses that had been established in the seventeenth century, lunatic wards were added both to workhouses and some voluntary hospitals. This growth of interest fostered four further developments. First, there was a growing legal concern over the manner in which people came to be incarcerated. Second, there was an equal concern over the conditions in which the inmates of such institutions were obliged to live. Third, there was a growing academic as well as lay interest in the nature of mental illness and mental retardation, and in the possibility that cures might be made. Fourth and finally, there developed new, specialised medical occupations. In other words, idiocy and lunacy began to become the subject of formal as well as lay methods of care; to become the concern of professionals as well as families and private entrepreneurs. In addition, there was increasing concern about the use of madhouses. As Patricia Allderidge, a medical historian, has pointed out, Acts such as that passed in 1774 were largely to allay people's fears that madhouses could be used as 'a handy receptacle for rich uncles, infatuated daughters, supernumerary wives, or spendthrift sons' (Allderidge, 1979, p.332). The Act required the licensing and inspection of private madhouses, the notification of all admissions, and the certification by a physician, surgeon or apothecary that the patient was in fact insane.

☐ What does this reveal concerning people's fears in this area?
■ First that some of the mad were themselves to be feared, and second that the certification of madness could be misused — that special guarantees were needed by those in a position of authority.

Such fears were not new: earlier laws had as one of their main concerns the fear that a person's enfeebled mental state might be exploited by others.

☐ The 1774 Act reflects a change in attitude from previous centuries concerning the nature of idiocy and lunacy. What was that change?
■ Supervision of the care of the mentally ill changed from being the responsibility of the courts to that of doctors. This change in responsibility was accompanied by a change in theories of mental disorder: supernatural explanations increasingly gave way to naturalistic explanations, and as the latter spread, so too did the involvement of doctors.

Public Health: uneven advance
The mixture of public and private provision which was a feature of care for the insane, was also true of other aspects of health care in the eighteenth century, including that of public health measures. Improvements were very uneven. In London, many streets in the City and West End were rebuilt according to more spacious standards, and when William Hutton, a native of Birmingham, visited London in 1785 he was astounded to find that

> besides many superb edifices, of a public and private nature, every street and passage in the whole city, and its environs, has been paved in one regular and convenient stile; an expence equal in value to the whole dominions of some sovereign princes ... (Cited in Buer, 1926, p.82)

No doubt he had not ventured across the 'whole city', however, for things were certainly not like this in the East

End or elsewhere. However, many English towns began, in Hutton's phrase, to follow 'London at a humble distance'. Between 1785 and 1800, 221 Acts of Paving and other Parochial Improvements were passed. Some of this improvement was funded by public subscription, the rest by rates. At the same time, there was also a great wave of building activity and many old parts of towns and cities were torn down and replaced. Some of the new replacement buildings included another product of the industrial revolution — the water-closet patented by Joseph Bramah in 1778.

Infectious diseases remained the greatest threat to health, including the much dreaded smallpox. Many historians have argued that the health care services of this period had little or no impact on mortality, indeed they may even have made things worse.* However, there is some evidence to suggest that, in the case of smallpox, inoculation was an effective measure. In the 1770s it was being widely used, both privately and publicly under the Poor Law provision. For example, a wealthy family of practitioners, the Suttons, claimed to have treated 300 000 people privately and offered free inoculation to the poor if the rest of the parish were treated. Daniel Sutton inoculated 417 poor people in one day in Maldon in Essex, perhaps using coercion, for in some places poor relief was refused to those who would not consent to the treatment. In other parts of Europe, smallpox inoculation was administered by the clergy. Robert Heller, a medical historian, has shown how in Roman Catholic France the rural clergy were told to urge their congregations to accept inoculation (Heller, 1976).

Although each country used different means to implement such public health measures, they all shared a common interest in improving and increasing the level of social regulation: much of Europe was experiencing long-term economic change and population growth, agricultural upheaval, and the continuous growth of towns. In England, particularly, the family's role in economic activity was being displaced by the factory system, and large numbers of dispossessed — paupers, beggars, vagrants and itinerant unemployed were being created.

Amidst these fundamental changes, the accumulation of numerical facts began on an enormous scale. As you have seen, the potential of statistics had been mapped out in the previous century. By the end of the eighteenth century the 'science of the state' was emerging as, in Hacking's words, 'a transnational industrial philosophy'. Statistics claimed not simply to be counting, but, as expressed in the preface to the 21-volume *Statistical Survey of Scotland* published in the 1790s, enquiring into 'the conditions of life of a country, in order to establish the *quantum of happiness* of the inhabitants'. By the early nineteenth century such surveys had taken on the appearance of obsessiveness, covering crime, suicide, illnesses, epidemics, in fact a desire to list all the numbers known to all humankind. This desire was not confined to northern Europe. The Russian writer, Alexander Herzen, exiled to Vyatka in Siberia between 1835 and 1838, reported:

> It so happened that the Ministry of the Interior had just been seized with a fit of statistics. Orders were issued that committees should be appointed all over the country ... to show a maximum and minimum as well as averages, and conclusions based on a comparison of ten years (for nine of which, if you please, no statistics at all had been recorded). (Herzen, 1980 edn, p.211)

That the notion of collecting statistics on all those topics could have spread so rapidly to the smallest villages of Siberia is an indication of the power of the mode of thought. But to implement this new approach, to regulate medicine and health, something more was needed: in England and Wales, there were no fewer than 15 000 parishes, the central unit of administration; Germany was split into 300 separate states; even in France, the supposed home of central state power, local rights and privileges dating back to the Middle Ages regularly blocked central rule. All this was to change.

---

*The effectiveness of health care during this period is discussed in greater detail in *The Health of Nations*, *ibid.*, Chapter 8 (U205 Book III).

Objectives for Chapter 3

When you have studied this chapter, you should be able to:

3.1 Describe sixteenth and seventeenth-century attitudes to the care of the poor, and the attempts by emergent nation-states to impose central authority on health care, such as the licensing of practitioners, introducing public health measures, and providing care for an increasing number of poor people.

3.2 Discuss how the commercial revolution in northern European states led to a shift in the location of the centre of medical thought and training, and to the involvement of private as well as public enterprise in the provision of such facilities as madhouses, water supplies, poor relief and voluntary hospitals.

3.3 Describe how the revolution in both natural and social science which commenced in the seventeenth century gave rise to fundamental changes in the provision of health care, such as the concentration of hospitals on caring for the sick and, through an awareness of the 'population', attempts at social regulation.

Questions for Chapter 3

1 (*Objective 3.1*) Writing of sixteenth and seventeenth-century England, the historian Peter Laslett has commented on an area of 'public health': '... the perpetual preoccupation of the authorities of that era, governmental and municipal, with the supply of food for the poor ... Hence the strict control of all dealings in breadstuffs and all handlers of them, especially buyers and sellers of wheat. The stocks of corn so conspicuous in the records of Tudor and Stuart London were examples of a policy which had to be pursued all the time and in deadly earnest' (Laslett, 1979, pp.124–5).

Does such a policy have parallels with the reasoning behind the Poor Law Acts around the end of the sixteenth century?

2 (*Objective 3.2*) In 1767 extraordinary scenes occurred in London involving Scottish medical practitioners and the College of Physicians: having 'organised themselves for direct action', the practitioners 'resolved to storm the College, and this they did, breaking windows and manhandling the servants of the College. Having broken down the hall door, [they] poured in and sat among the College fellows then in session ...' (Hamilton, 1981, p.142).

What circumstances might have explained these scenes?

3 (*Objective 3*) In a lecture in 1676, William Petty noted how: 'another cause of defect in the art of medicine and consequently of its contempt is that there have not been hospitals for the accommodation of sick people' (cited in Woodward, 1974, p.7).

In 1754, Benjamin Franklin, describing the need for a voluntary hospital in Philadelphia, wrote: 'how expensive the providing good and careful nurses, and other attendants for want whereof many must suffer greatly and some probably perish that might otherwise have been restored to health and comfort, and become useful to themselves, their families, and the publick for many years after' (cited in Rosen, 1963, p.23).

What factors contributed to the establishment of hospitals which were specifically for the sick?

4

1800–1939: an age of reform

The period dealt with in this chapter (1800–1939) saw many major changes in all aspects of health care and society. The chapter necessarily is long. To help you through it, it has been subdivided into three sections: 1800–1860, 1860–1913 and 1913–1939. Remember that you are expected to acquire from the material a familiarity with the main developments, not a long list of dates. Refer to the chapter objectives before and during your study of the text if you are unsure about what you are expected to learn.

From this foul drain the greatest stream of human industry flows out to fertilize the whole world. From this filthy sewer pure gold flows. Here humanity attains its most complete development and its most brutish, here civilisation works its miracles and civilised man is turned almost into a savage. (de Tocqueville (edited Mayer), 1958, p.107)

Alexis de Tocqueville's description of Manchester in 1835 could equally well have applied to any of the other newly industrialised towns and cities of Britain. What was so striking to the visiting French aristocrat was the contrast between the immense wealth that industrialisation was producing and the appalling conditions in which the mass of the population were living. More and more people were packed into the central areas of cities, which often lacked even the most basic sanitation, the back streets were constantly strewn with human excrement, and drinking water was drawn from polluted canals and rivers. The River Ayre, which received waste from Leeds, Bradford, Keighley, Skipton, Halifax, Huddersfield and Wakefield, was described in 1840 as:

a reservoir of poison carefully kept for the purpose of breeding a pestilence in the town ... full of refuse from water closets, cesspools, privies, common drains, dunghill drainage, infirmary refuse, waste from slaughter houses, chemical soaps, gas, dyehouses and manufacturers; coloured by blue and black dyes, pig manure, old urine wash; there were dead animals, vegetable substances and occasionally a decomposed human body. (Cited in Wohl, 1983, p.235)

The inadequacy of public health measures to combat the worsening environmental conditions was matched by the failure of personal health care to have any significant effect. Early nineteenth-century medicine lacked both the means and the organisation to cure diseases. The Royal College of Physicians contained fewer than 200 members and refused fully to recognise Scottish medical degrees. The ecclesiastical licensing system for midwives had completely broken down; the profession, such as it was, was in a state of anarchy. Nursing was in no better condition. The classic picture of what contemporary nursing could sometimes mean is Charles Dickens' portrayal in *Martin Chuzzlewit* of Sairey Gamp: '"Mrs Harris" I says, "leave the bottle on the chimney-piece, and don't ask me to take none, but let me put my lips to it when I am so disposed"' (Dickens, 1844, Chap. 19). The voluntary hospitals could cope with only a few thousand in-patients, and conditions in some of the workhouse infirmaries were the subject of repeated scandal.

In many ways, the early decades of the nineteenth century were marked by a deterioration in the state of health of the majority of the population as the new dangers associated with industrialisation and urbanisation were added to the long-standing hazards of poor nutrition and infectious diseases. Industrial diseases were simply an accepted part of working life, as inevitable and as unpleasant as the long hours and conditions of employment. Miner's asthma or 'black spit', potter's asthma, or 'potter's rot', brass founder's ague, matchmaker's necrosis or 'phossy jaw', and chimney sweep's cancer or 'soot wart' were just some of the diseases that were a part of nineteenth-century vocabulary. There can have been few industrial workers who were free of respiratory disease. Gradually, however, this began to change, so that by the beginning of the twentieth century the state of people's health in Britain had improved. How did this come about?

First, social structures were being transformed both by industrial and political changes. The historian Eric Hobsbawm has captured these transformations in the following way:

> Words are witnesses which often speak louder than documents. Let us consider a few English words which were invented, or gained their modern meanings, substantially in this period ... 'industry', 'industrialist', 'factory', 'middle class', 'working class', 'capitalism' and 'socialism'. They include 'aristocracy' as well as 'railway', 'liberal' and 'conservative' as political terms, 'nationality', 'scientist', and 'engineer', 'proletariat' and (economic) 'crisis'. 'Utilitarian' and 'statistics', 'sociology' and several other names of modern sciences, 'journalism' and 'ideology' are all coinages or adaptations of this period. So are 'strike' and 'pauperism'. To imagine the modern world without these words (i.e. without the things and concepts for which they provide names) is to measure the profundity of the revolution which broke out between 1789 and 1848 ... this revolution has transformed and continues to transform, the entire world. (Hobsbawm, 1962, p.17)

Second, progress was being made in science and technology. Although this had little impact on personal health care before the end of the nineteenth century, the application of science to the study of the health of the population, by new social survey and epidemiological methods, assisted in the enactment of public health legislation.

A third factor, that of the fear of epidemics, had both an immediate and a long term influence. The cholera epidemics in the mid-nineteenth century resurrected the spectre of the Black Death throughout Europe. The epidemics aroused concern in both middle and working classes, although their worst effects were felt amongst the poor and this contributed to the passage of key public health legislation, which was to produce widespread benefits.

And, finally, underlying all these factors, were industrial growth and rising living standards, which, especially in the second half of the nineteenth century, provided the means to improve health through better nutrition, housing, clothing, and investment in public health institutions and other health care services.

1800–1860

At the beginning of the nineteenth century, over one in ten of the population was on poor relief and by 1815 the workhouses — now 4 000 in number — contained more than 100 000 paupers. Amid widespread poverty, appalling housing, dangerous working conditions and the frequent absence of sanitation, epidemic diseases like typhoid and cholera, and endemic diseases like tuberculosis, all thrived. England, being first to industrialise, was also first to develop a social philosophy expressly attuned to an industrial society. Essentially, what was at issue were the respective roles of *the market* and *the state*.

☐ Had the state tried to intervene in pre-industrial England?

■ Yes, in many ways, including attempts to appoint sewage inspectors and regulate the practice of physicians.

By the late eighteenth century, however, all this was being ferociously criticised. The only way to let industrialisation proceed unimpeded, it was argued, was to sweep away all the ancient obstacles and restrictions to the operation of free markets — for the pursuit of economic self-interest would result in the advancement of the interests of society as a whole. Adam Smith, the eighteenth-century Scottish economist and one of the chief architects of this philosophy, had argued that the state should confine its activities to just three areas: (i) security against foreign enemies, (ii) the administration of justice, and (iii) the carrying out of tasks that were in the interest of the community but that would not be undertaken solely through profit motive. This last category was the one in which the arguments over providing health care, public health measures and poor relief were fought. If left to the market, would the provision of these services be in the best interest of society, or would the government have to have systematic policies?

In the early years of the nineteenth century, the need for state involvement in poor relief was widely accepted. Indeed, the provision of relief had even been extended to those who had work but were still in poverty. Legally sanctioned in 1796, the cost of such provision had grown rapidly. By 1818, leading economists of the day, such as Thomas Malthus, were arguing that this way lay national ruin and calling for a complete reversal of policy. The 1834 Poor Law Amendment Act embodied the view that relief provided for the poor, sick, aged and infirm by local or central government should be reduced to the bare minimum. The cardinal principle was to *deter*. It was essential that poverty be made painful, by discipline and by ensuring that relief raised no one in receipt of it to the level of the lowest-paid labourers. This was the principle of 'less eligibility', and is still resurrected in political debates over social security and unemployment benefits.

In order to implement this policy of deterrence, *centralisation* was necessary, for if the central government did not have control, local governments might continue to provide morsels of generosity. In consequence, the existing administrative units of local government — mainly parishes — were amalgamated and radically reduced in number from 15 000 units to fewer than 600 Poor Law Unions, each administered by Boards of Guardians answerable to three national Poor Law Commissioners. The Boards of Guardians were to be elected, though at this time few people had the vote.

☐ What flaws can you detect in the assumptions underlying the principles of deterrence and centralisation?

■ Deterrence assumed that poverty was an individual moral weakness, rather than a consequence of sickness, handicap, old age or the workings of the economic system. Centralisation assumed that the central administrative apparatus was sufficiently well developed to coordinate, check and exercise control over the almost 600 elected Poor Law Unions.

The fact was that deterrence could not create employment for the unemployed when no work existed, nor could it cure the ill-health and sickness that resulted from shocking living conditions. In this sense the philosophy of the Poor Law Amendment Act was fundamentally mistaken. Within a few years of the passing of the Poor Law Amendment Act, the secretary to the three Commissioners, the lawyer Edwin

Chadwick, had decided that deterrence was not enough. The report of the Commissioners in 1840 stated why this conclusion had been reached:

All epidemics, and all infectious diseases, are attended with charges, immediate and ultimate, on the poor rates. Labourers are suddenly thrown, by infectious diseases, into a state of destitution, for which immediate relief must be given. In the case of death, the widow and the children are thrown as paupers on the parish. The amount of poverty thus produced is frequently so great as to render it good economy on the part of the administrators of the Poor Law to incur the charges for preventing the evils where they are attributable to physical causes. (Cited in Eckstein, 1958, p.13)

☐ How would you describe the grounds on which this argument is based?

■ The appeal is for prevention on the grounds of economy.

While the Poor Law Commissioners in Britain were defending the need for the involvement of a strong central government in the provision of social assistance, in other more economically backward parts of Europe a more radical solution to poverty was being called for. One of the foremost advocates of such an approach was Rudolf Virchow, a young doctor who was later to become one of the great figures of nineteenth-century biomedicine. Reporting for the Prussian government on a massive outbreak of typhoid in the poor and largely Polish-speaking province of Upper Silesia in 1848, he concluded that:

it is no longer a question of the medical treatment and care of this or that person taken ill with typhoid, but the well-being of one and a half million citizens who find themselves at the lowest level of moral and physical decline. With one and a half million of people you cannot begin with palliatives, you have to be radical. If you want to intercede in Upper Silesia, you must start by inciting the population to united effort. Education, freedom and welfare can never be fully attained from the outside, in the manner of a present, but from the people's realization of their real needs. As far as I can see, it is only by calling for the national reorganization of Upper Silesia that the presently apathetic and exhausted people could bring about their own rebirth. (In Taylor and Rieger, 1984, p.206)

☐ What, according to Virchow, was the only means of improving the people's health?

■ Political reorganisation of the state had to be pursued by the people themselves: solutions could not be imposed, and medical treatment without wider change would be no more than a palliative.

Virchow's analysis — still a radical position in debates about health care today — led him to support strongly the German 'middle-class revolution' of 1848, which called for far-reaching changes to allow Germany to industrialise and catch up with Britain. That revolution was not immediately successful, but it did place a range of issues on the political agenda. In Germany and elsewhere, these could only be ignored at risk of further revolutionary agitation. The result was a long period of reform of health care services for the poor and the gradual establishment of more effective public health measures.

The doctors employed by Poor Law Unions began both to expand in number, and to take on new duties. By 1838 there were 1 830 medical officers, by 1845 there were 2 680. These doctors and other reformers began to draw attention to the conditions of the sick in the workhouses, and to campaign for improvements. When, admidst a raging smallpox epidemic, the Vaccination Acts of 1840 and 1841 were passed, allowing free vaccination to all, the Poor Law medical officers were the only people organised on a national basis who were able to implement mass vaccination. In 1842, 378 000 children were vaccinated, and deaths fell from 10 000 in 1840 to 2 700. This was the first occasion on which free medical attention had been dispensed nationally by government. Despite the fact that personal health care for the sick poor had been given hardly more than a passing mention in the Poor Law Amendment Act, medical services provided through the Act became more elaborate throughout the nineteenth century, eventually forming the basis of state-provided medical care

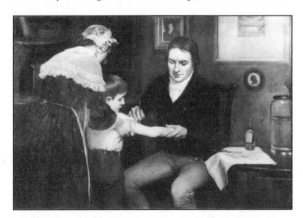

Figure 4.1 Edward Jenner, shown here in a painting by E. Board, performing his first smallpox vaccination in 1796 on a country boy named James Phipps. When Jenner's findings were published in 1798, Napoleon at once had his troops vaccinated, and Thomas Jefferson established its acceptance in the United States by having his family vaccinated in 1801. But opposition was widespread, particularly in England, where the Society of Anti-Vaccinationists (founded in 1798) was active.

and paving the way for the introduction of the National Health Service. This forward look suggests therefore that the 1834 Act did not work as its designers had intended.

Chadwick ran a ceaseless campaign to counter the effects of pauperism by means of public health measures. He was a skilful propagandist, and also made use of the latest research methods, such as those pioneered by the French doctor, Louis-René Villermé. (In 1826 Villermé published a study of mortality in different districts of Paris that pointed to a definite relationship between poverty and disease. Two years later he demonstrated how mortality rates were closely related to the living conditions of the different social classes.) Using data submitted by Poor Law medical officers, Chadwick published in 1842 a 'Report ... on the Sanitary Conditions of the Labouring Population of Great Britain'. It was to prove to be the single most important event in the establishment, only six years later, of the first national public health legislation and a new central authority.

While Chadwick championed many public health measures, such as the need for attention to housing conditions and overcrowding and to the health hazards associated with poor working conditions, it was to sanitation that he directed most of his attention. For Chadwick, effective prevention of disease would only come about if sewage and other filth were removed from the streets, clean water provided and adequate ventilation ensured. This view rested upon the contemporary theory that most epidemic disease was due to bad smells and gases known as miasmas. It is interesting to note that the failure correctly to identify the cause of infectious diseases did not impede the effectiveness of the preventive measures that were taken.

☐ Can you recall any previous examples where effective intervention *preceded* accurate understanding of the cause of a disease?

■ The classic example is that of John Snow and cholera, in which an outbreak of the disease was controlled by his removing the handle of the water pump in Broad Street, London at a time when the cause was still unknown. Another example is that of pernicious anaemia, the cause of which is still not fully understood, yet effective therapy has been available for over 50 years.*

*The example of Snow and cholera is discussed in Open University (1985) *Studying Health and Disease*, The Open University Press (U205 Book I) and that of pernicious anaemia appears in Loudon, Irvine, 'The history of pernicious anaemia from 1822 to the present day' in Black, N. *et al* (1985) *Health and Disease: a Reader*, Open University Press (U205 Course Reader), and in *Medical Knowledge: Doubt and Certainty*, ibid. (U205 Book II).

Chadwick recommended that single local authorities should be established to administer all sanitary matters with both expert medical advice (from a full time Medical Officer of Health) and engineering advice. At the centre he argued there should be a Central Board of Health directing and advising. His report was well received, and in 1848 after a great deal of controversy the first British Public Health Act was passed. There were, however, two major problems — the provision of adequate sanitation and water supplies was very expensive, and also it was relatively easy for towns to avoid taking any action as the legislation was only permissive, that is it simply *permitted* towns to establish the public health measures rather than *obliged* them to. Indeed, the measures in both this and a second Act in 1854 could only be applied with the support of two-thirds of the property owners and ratepayers, or if the crude mortality rate was above 23 per 1 000. In practice, a lack both of central state control and powers of coercion, in combination with the intricacies of the law and the voluntary nature of the legislation, seriously delayed much sanitary reform before the 1860s. The sort of local political struggles that permissive legislation gave rise to can be seen in what took place in Bala in North Wales following the 1858 Local Government Act:

> Earlier that month the ratepayers of Bala had held a properly convened public meeting at which they had decided, with only one dissenting voice, to petition the government to be brought under the 1858 Local Government Act. This would enable the ratepayers to establish a Local Board of Health, to cleanse the town, provide it with sewers and with clean water, light it and generally help to create conditions that would make it a more salubrious and comfortable place to live in. The odd man out in this movement was Richard Price ... the proprietor of an estate of 9 000 acres, one of the richest landowners, chairman of the bench and the most powerful man in what local government existed. He explained, 'that there does not exist within the said Town any occasion for the said Act, owing to the poverty of the inhabitants and the small amount of rateable Property'. Later on, he gave it as his opinion that the whole movement was nothing but a conspiracy on the part of a few people in the town, 'merely to get the management of the place into their own hands'. (Jones, 1979, p.5)

Similar problems arose with the implementation of legislation to control the appalling conditions in mines and factories, particularly for children. The first of these, in 1802, stipulated that children should work no more than twelve hours a day, do no night work, and that the place of work should be ventilated and twice a year washed down. Subsequent legislation set the minimum working age in cotton mills at nine, but made it incumbent upon parents, and not the mill owners, to ensure their children were not under age. In practice, the first legislation to achieve any progress was the Factories Act of 1833, which established the Factory Inspectorate. Initially this had only four members and it was not until the end of the century that legislation required 'certifying surgeons' to investigate cases of industrial disease and 'appointed surgeons' to undertake the regular medical examination of workers in specified industries. (The first Medical Inspector of Factories was not to be appointed until 1898.)

Doctors and nurses: steps to reform

The most visible aspects of the Industrial Revolution may have been the conditions of the poor in the ever-swelling towns and cities, but the middle classes were also growing, and as they grew they also exerted influences on the development of health care.

Both middle and upper classes by and large continued to receive formal care in their own homes, but the middle classes could not afford the very high fees set both by the physicians and the élite surgeons of the voluntary hospitals. What they wanted was a reasonably cheap but reliable service. They also wanted a doctor who was skilled across a variety of areas, a generalist such as those being produced in very large numbers by the Scottish medical schools where the division between surgeons and apothecaries no longer existed.

Such *general practitioners* (GPs), as they were labelled by the 1820s, were defined as 'ordinary attendants in private life', in contrast to *consultants* who were of superior rank and acted as 'extraordinary advisers in difficult cases', though another commentator added 'that consultants are sought in cases of less urgency among those who have the advantages of ease and affluence' (cited in Waddington, 1985, p.17). Such definitions of the GP and consultant could hardly be bettered today, though it is important to note that at that time, given the relatively small number of hospitals, some GPs also acted as consultants, advising their colleagues on the more difficult cases, particularly outside the cities and large towns.

In addition to the development of generalists, several other changes took place in the provision of formal care that demanded a radical revision of the organisation of medical practice. The divisions of the Colleges, Companies and Societies no longer suited such developments: thousands of surgeons were still excluded from membership of the Royal Colleges, and those physicians with Scottish degrees were not fully recognised by the Royal College of Physicians. In addition, the state was employing increasing numbers of doctors as superintendents at the new asylums for the insane (which will be discussed shortly), as Medical Officers of Health with local authorities, and as Poor Law doctors. The range of qualifications of those employed for these posts illustrates the piecemeal manner in which medical training had developed over the previous centuries (Table 4.1).

Indeed, some local authorities and Poor Law Unions felt that doctors had no special qualifications for these posts, and appointed lay people, sometimes on the basis of the lowest tender. Doctoring could still be a poverty-stricken and humiliating business. There were stories of Poor Law doctors ending up in the same workhouses at which they had once worked.

□ Who, apart from the ordinary practitioners, do you think would have desired reform of medical training and practice?

■ The state, which was increasingly involved in activities such as vaccination campaigns and the collection of statistics, and was increasingly important as an employer.

Chadwick was an advocate of reform in this area, too, arguing that:

The multiplication ... of such fragmentitious professional services is injurious to the public and the profession ... by multiplying the poor, ill-paid and ill-conditioned medical men. (1842 Report, cited in Hodgkinson, 1967, p.633)

Faced with a similar situation, France undertook systematic reform early in the century, producing a unified profession with a national register and a common basic training for all doctors.

By 1830, Paris had thirty specialised teaching hospitals, containing 20 000 patients and providing clinical training for 5 000 students. In France, too, attempts were made to create a new class of medical practitioner to deal with the medical problems of the poor — the 'health officer'. Health officers were also to be properly trained, but far more quickly and at a far more basic level. The initial version of the health officer did not in fact survive long. In Belgium, for example, the grade only lasted from 1803 to 1835, at which point it was abolished. The idea, however, was to survive in other ways: in Russia, with the creation later in the century of the 'feldsher'; and in the Third World in more recent times, as you will see later.

None the less, in most western European countries doctoring was soon to be the preserve of the university-trained. Britain was no exception, but the fight was long and hard. On one side, bitterly opposing any change, were the Royal Colleges and the Society of Apothecaries. On the other side were a great variety of doctors and reformers. New tactics were adopted during the conflict: rank and file doctors were one of the earliest occupations to embrace industrial trade unionism in order to control the conditions under which they laboured — eventually with great success. The *British Medical Journal*, the mass-circulation organ of the new trade union, the British Medical Association (BMA) (formed in 1832), was first published in 1857. But membership of the BMA was to remain low until the early twentieth century, and it was another medical mass-circulation journal, *The Lancet*, founded in 1823, that led the most vigorous campaign for reform. Thomas Wakley, the editor of *The Lancet*, in 1831 led some three or four hundred ordinary surgeons, most of them probably GPs, into the Royal College of Surgeons, from whose discussions they were normally barred, and held an emergency meeting. After a violent struggle, Wakley was eventually removed by the police, or Bow Street Runners as they were then called.

It was another twenty-seven years before the General Medical Act of 1858 reformed the tangle of occupations and training. The Act (it had taken sixteen attempts to pass it) abolished the three ancient professions of physicians, surgeons and apothecaries and replaced them with two new professions: pharmacists and a single, united medical profession. The latter was to receive a basic university training in all the relevant sciences as well as systematic voluntary training in hospitals which were designated as suitable for teaching. At the same time, and just as important, all those who had not been trained were driven out of the market, a measure that limited still further the opportunity for women to be practitioners.

The principal remaining role for women in formal care was nursing, which was also reformed in the mid-nineteenth century. Look at the illustration from the *Nursing Record* of 1888 and the way it contrasts nurses of that year with their predecessors of 50 years before (Figure 4.2 overleaf).

Table 4.1 The qualifications of Poor Law Medical Officers in 1836

Description	Number	Per cent
Physicians only	9	0.5
Licentiate apothecaries only	316	17
Surgeons only	294	16
Surgeons and apothecaries	914	50
Other apothecaries	201	11
Army/navy surgeons	29	2
Unqualified	27	1
Others	40	2
Total	1830	100

(Source: Hodgkinson, 1967, Table 2.1, p.69)

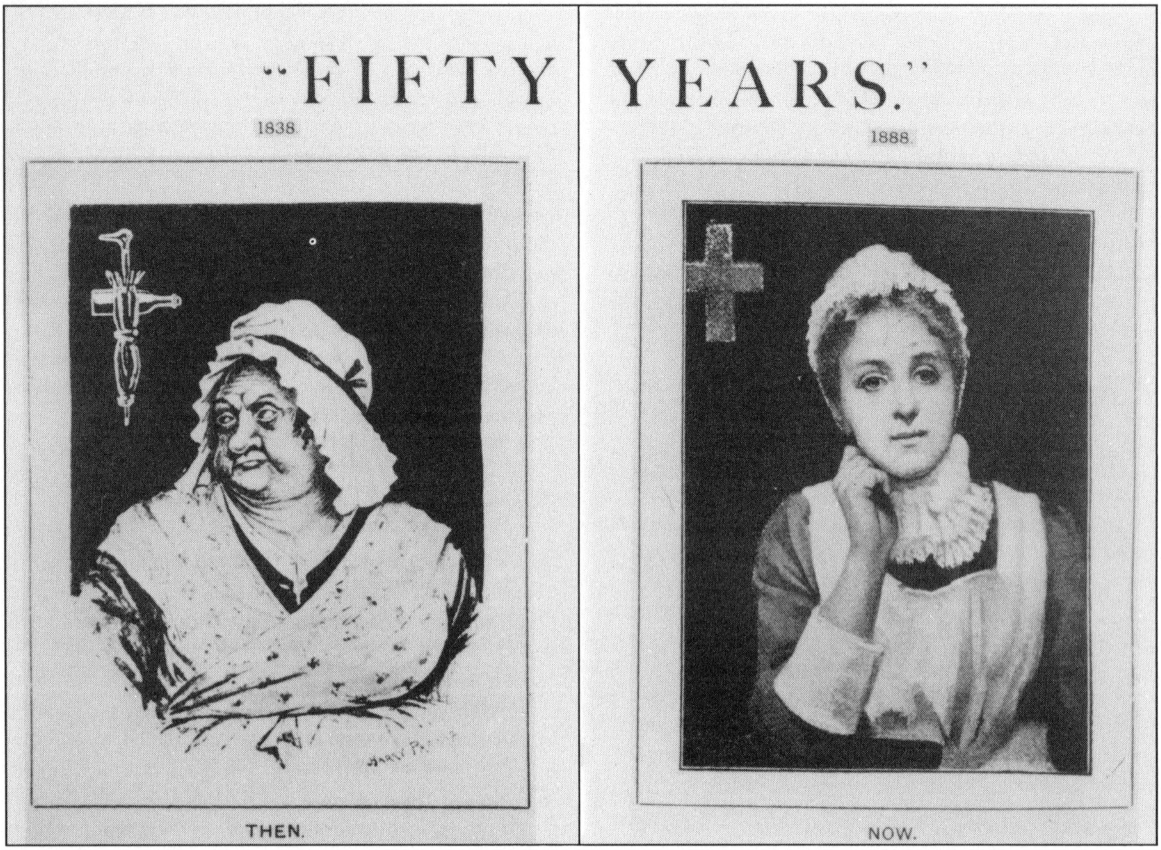

Figure 4.2 'Then' and 'Now': images of nurses in 1838 and in 1888.

□   What differences are there in the way nurses were portrayed in 1888 and in 1838?

■   The nurse in 1838 is old, dirty, plump and ugly, dressed as a 'downstairs' servant — one who would not be allowed to undertake duties in the public part of the house. The picture shows her shiftily avoiding the viewer's gaze. By contrast the nurse in 1888 is young, clean, slender and pretty, dressed as an 'upstairs' servant, and fit to be seen by visitors to the house. She looks directly at the viewer. Notice, too, the symbols in the top left-hand corner of each picture. In 1838, there was a gin bottle and an umbrella or 'gamp' (intended to recall Dickens' Sairey Gamp). By 1888 this has given way to the cross, evoking Christian charity and devotion.

How had this transformation come about? The first influences compelling changes in nursing came both from France and from Germany. In post-revolutionary France, the reorganisation of the hospitals brought large numbers of patients before doctors, who were developing new ways

of extending their knowledge by means of direct observations in life and post-mortem examination in death. By the first decade of the nineteenth century these innovations, the basis of modern medical practice, were spreading across Europe, along with the new or rediscovered instruments for making or calibrating observations, including the stethoscope, pulse watch and thermometer. Developments in science and technology were transforming not only the practice of medicine but also health care occupations and institutions.

At first, all of these tools were used solely by doctors. The natural history of diseases was charted to form the basis of the classifications which are still used today.* By mid century, the major categories were reasonably well delineated. The frontier of discovery had moved on and medical interest was shifting towards using this knowledge

---

*The development of the classification of disease (*nosology*) is discussed in *Studying Health and Disease*, *ibid*. (U205 Book I) and *Medical Knowledge: Doubt and Certainty*, *ibid*. (U205 Book II).

in a search for better therapies. Patient care was now more a matter of identifying the presence of a disease whose natural history would be predictable. It was an uneconomic and uninteresting use of doctors' time simply to observe progress, although it was increasingly important to know when particular things were happening so that appropriate interventions could be made.

There was, then, a need for a reliable observer who could observe patients and notify the doctor when his contribution was required. This would have to be a person who was both sufficiently educated and reasonably conscientious, but who was willing to accept a subordinate

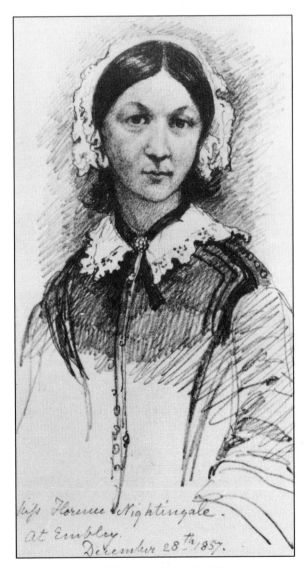

Figure 4.3 Portrait of Florence Nightingale, 1857.

role. One way of filling that role was developed in Germany. In 1833 the Protestant Deaconesses Institute was founded in Kaiserworth in the Rhineland. It combined two crucial ideas: first, that of systematic nurse training, and second, that of a strong religious vocation. In 1851, it was visited by a young, unmarried, upper-class English woman — Florence Nightingale — who had scandalised her family by announcing her intention to train as a nurse. As an extract from her diary written at the age of 31 reveals, she had not been happy with her daily round:

> O heavy days — oh evenings that seem never to end — and for how many years have I watched that drawing-room clock and thought it never would reach ten! and for twenty, thirty, years more to do this! ... Women don't consider themselves as human beings at all. There is absolutely no God, no country, no duty to them at all except family ... I have known a good deal of convents ... But I know nothing surpasses the petty grinding tyranny of a good English family. And the only salvation is that the tyrannized submits with a heart full of affection. (Cited in Woodham-Smith, 1951, pp.62–3)

Such dissatisfactions drove other upper-class women of this period, both in Europe and the USA, to fight to enable women to seek an active career as doctors. But Nightingale concentrated her energies on the reform of nursing. Somewhat similar developments were taking place elsewhere in Europe, but Nightingale had perhaps the most profound influence of all. The specific impetus was the Crimean War and the enormous casualties which this produced. Beginning in 1853 with, on the one side, France and Britain, and on the other, Russia, the armies suffered more from the assaults of typhus and 'hospital fever' than they ever did from military action.

On the Russian side, the military surgeon Nikolai Pirogoff began to instigate nursing reform. On the British side, the domestic outcry at reports of the appalling conditions provided Nightingale with the perfect opportunity to put ideas into practice. Along with forty other nurses, she arrived at the military hospital at Scutari on the outskirts of Constantinople (modern-day Istanbul) in the winter of 1854. The British Army was in a state of administrative and military chaos, and medical services were almost non-existent. Casualties were being shipped across the Black Sea on a two to three week voyage from the Crimean peninsula to a huge barrack-house at Scutari. The death rate on this journey was reported at 74 per 1 000, but in the filthy and crowded barrack hospital it rose to a staggering 420 per 1 000. Nightingale acted decisively, reforming the food, cleaning, laundry, water, sanitation, finances, transport and purchasing policy of the hospital.

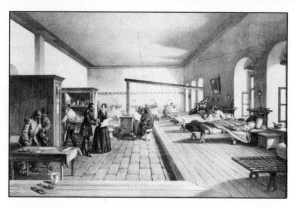

Figure 4.4 One of the wards in the hospital at Scutari after Nightingale's reforms had transformed conditions. Lithograph by E. Walker after W. Simpson, 1856.

This brought her into constant conflict with the Army medical authorities and administrators. However, extraordinary public support and financial backing in Britain enabled her to effect the changes she wanted. The image of the 'lady with the lamp', the ministering angel of mercy, of wounded men kissing her shadow, sprang directly from the fact that basic amenities were being provided regularly for ordinary soldiers for the first time. The mortality rate fell dramatically to 22 per 1000. A commemorative brooch, designed by Prince Albert, and presented as 'a mark of the high approbation of your Sovereign', was for many years worn by nurses in Britain.

Nightingale spent a relatively short amount of her long life directly involved in nursing: after Scutari she turned to hospital reform, public health and the need for change in the Empire-wide Army Medical Service. But her work at Scutari had two major consequences: first, she secularised nursing, removing from it the last vestiges of religious control; second, she popularised nursing as a respectable job for respectable women. Her influence and work is still controversial, as you will see shortly. Nevertheless, the 1850s marked a watershed after which nursing was to develop national qualifications, elaborate training structures, mass-circulation journals, and nationwide methods of occupational organisation.

Hospitals, workhouses and asylums

A major influence on developments in doctoring and nursing was the very rapid growth of hospitals in Britain in the first half of the nineteenth century. These hospitals fell into three broad categories: the voluntary hospitals, whose origins were discussed in the previous chapter, the workhouse infirmaries, and the asylums.

In 1800 there were probably around 400–500 beds in the

voluntary hospitals of England; by 1861 this had grown to almost 11 000. The money for this expansion came largely from public bequests and charitable donations, and was directed by doctors into the formation of hospital *medical schools*; such doctors increasingly saw the voluntary hospital as a way of providing teaching and research material. By 1861 around 40 per cent of all beds in the voluntary sector were in teaching hospitals; in London the figure was nearer 80 per cent.

Insofar as it is possible to generalise about such a disparate collection of institutions, the following trends were evident in the voluntary hospitals during this period: first, the people admitted were overwhelmingly the poor. In 1861, the census indicated that only 157 of the 10 414 inmates were in 'professional' occupations. Second, the voluntary hospitals were increasingly picking and choosing their admissions, such that few children, chronic cases, infectious disease cases or paupers were admitted, but more acute cases were.

> ☐ What reasons can you think of for this?
> ■ Acute cases were short-stay and chronic cases long-stay. Acute cases therefore provided more teaching material, and more cases treated for each bed bequeathed, making donations easier to attract.

Third, as attention focused more on acute care and on teaching, so voluntary hospital out-patient departments started to grow. Among the reasons for this were that out-patient departments were a good way of selecting teaching material for admission, and that they swelled in an inexpensive way the number of cases a hospital could report having treated in its appeals and annual statements: such 'performance indicators' were important in the competition to attract funds. Whatever the reasons, the trend accelerated later in the century, with implications to which we will return later.

Finally, the established voluntary hospitals stuck to their traditions as *general hospitals*: that is, they were increasingly concentrating on acute work, but not specialising within acute care. The pressure towards specialisation therefore resulted in new *specialist hospitals*: eye hospitals (nineteen founded outside London between 1808 and 1832), children's hospitals, obstetric hospitals, and so on. In London alone, four new special hospitals opened in the 1830s, seven in the 1840s, eight in the 1850s, and sixteen in the 1860s.

The voluntary hospitals, therefore, were doing more work in some areas, but withdrawing from others. The cases they refused had to be taken up by the *workhouse* (or *Poor Law*) *infirmaries*.

Even in 1800, there were probably more beds in workhouse infirmaries than in voluntary hospitals. By 1843 there were 10 000; by 1861 the figure had soared to around

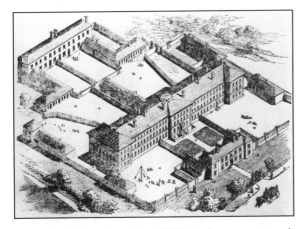

Figure 4.5 By amalgamating 15 000 local government administrative units into less than 600 Poor Law Unions it was possible to construct larger workhouse infirmaries. This new workhouse, opened on 4 August 1849, was for the United Parishes of Fulham and Hammersmith.

50 000, or almost five beds for every one in a voluntary hospital. Public provision, almost by default, had become the norm in hospital care.

As the voluntary hospitals increasingly refused to accept patients with chronic conditions or infectious diseases, and in a context of epidemics of smallpox and other infections repeatedly affecting the inhabitants of industrial cities, it became apparent to some that the standards of care and resources available to workhouse infirmaries would have to be improved. In 1866, *The Lancet*, in true campaigning tradition, published the results of its own enquiries into workhouses in London:

> How comes it that the public ... and the profession ... have nearly ignored these *real hospitals of the land*, while lavishing princely munificence on the splendid institutions [the voluntary hospitals] which ostensibly supply the national hospital requirements ... [but only] lightly touch the surface of the wide

field of London misery? (Cited in Hodgkinson, 1967, p.472)

The third category of hospitals, the *asylum*, changed rapidly in the first half of the nineteenth century; indeed, the whole notion of mental illness changed. At the beginning of the century there were two main types of institution dealing *exclusively* with the mentally ill. First, there were *private madhouses*, engaged in the 'madness business' as profit-making concerns. Subject to licensing and inspection since 1774 either by members of the Royal College of Physicians (in London) or by local magistrates (outside London), these 'licensed houses' grew rapidly in number from 45 in 1807 to 139 by 1844. Some, such as Ticehurst near Tunbridge Wells, were small, well-staffed, and catered almost exclusively for the London upper class or aristocracy. Many more dealt with paupers, packing in large numbers in order to show some profit. As Table 4.2 shows, by 1844 these private licensed houses contained about 5 000 patients. The second type of institution was the *county asylum*. Since 1808 it had been permissible to build asylums at county expense, but few counties had chosen to do so, and by 1844 the number of patients in such institutions, at around 4 500, was fewer than in the private madhouses.

The fact was that, at the time, the idea that the mad should be separated from society and treated in special institutions was not commonly accepted. The mentally ill either remained with their families or were found places in the workhouse along with the other old, sick, homeless or pauperised inmates.

However, new ideas about asylums had been circulating and gathering support since the late eighteenth century. After a scandal in the asylum in York, a wealthy Quaker merchant, William Tuke, had supported the founding of a new type of institution, called the *Retreat*. Opened in 1792, the Retreat was run on 'family lines'. The idea was to provide specialist care, to separate the mad from others and then to attempt systematic treatment — 'moral treatment', as Tuke called it. This institution attracted national and international attention, and became the model for reformers.

Table 4.2 Mid nineteenth-century asylum statistics

	Patients in asylums in					
	1844		1860		1870	
Institution	Number	%	Number	%	Number	%
Provincial licensed houses	3 346	30	2 356	10	2 204	6
Metropolitan licensed houses	1 827	16	1 944	8	2 700	8
County and Borough asylums	4 489	40	17 432	73	27 890	79
Others	1 610	14	1 985	8	2 369	7
Total	11 272	100	23 717	100	35 163	100

(Source: based on Scull; 1979, Tables 3 and 4, pp.190 and 193)

The outcome was the Lunatic Asylums Act, passed in 1845, which compelled every county and borough in England and Wales to provide accommodation in asylums for all pauper lunatics. Many acted promptly, others were prodded by the Lunacy Commissioners that the Act had also appointed. The results are clearly visible in Table 4.2: in fifteen years the number of patients in County and Borough asylums almost quadrupled.

Where had the people filling these new asylums come from? Partly, they were people previously held in the workhouses or gaols, private madhouses or in the homes of family or relatives. But look at Figure 4.6, which shows the official *rate of insanity* in England and Wales over this period.

☐ Between 1844 and 1860 what happened to the rate of insanity?

■ It rose from 12.66 per 10 000 to 19.12 per 10 000.

☐ What different explanations can you think of for this increase?

■ There are three possible explanations: first, that this represented a real growth in the amount of insanity in the population; second, that a large part of this was an *artefact* — the collection of statistics was poor in the first half of the century and so, perhaps was medical diagnosis; third, that the increase represented a major shift in the community's capacity or willingness to tolerate disturbed behaviour.

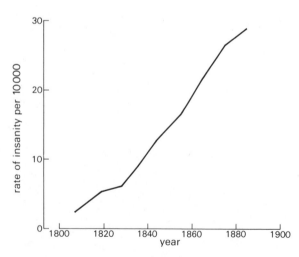

Figure 4.6 The numbers of persons officially identified as insane (including those in workhouses and the community) in England and Wales 1807–1885 per 10 000 population.
(Source: data derived from Table 8 in Scully, 1979, p.224)

All three arguments may have something in them, though the American historical sociologist, Andrew Scull, has argued largely in favour of the last explanation. Asylums created both an alternative to family care and the possibility of defining insanity far more broadly than hitherto — something particularly relevant to a rapidly urbanising society whose traditional culture and family obligations were under serious strain.

The reformers who had supported the 1845 Act had envisaged the new asylums as kindly, homely places, modelled on the Retreat at York. Their hopes were not realised, however: between 1830 and 1930 the average size of British asylums increased more than ten-fold, from just over 100 to more than 1 000. (In the USA some institutions went far higher, some even reaching 15 000 in the twentieth century.)

Faced with this vast expansion in size, and slowly realising that the reformers had overstated the possibility that the asylums would *cure* patients, local authorities sought ways to cut costs. As a result standards fell rapidly. Two years after it had opened in 1858, the Littlemore Asylum in Oxford charged eleven shillings a week to the parishes for each patient. By 1861 the magistrates who ran it had succeeded in reducing this to eight shillings, and two years later, despite rising prices for provisions and higher wages for staff, this had been further reduced. Asylums were increasingly becoming merely places of confinement. Indeed, some nineteenth-century psychiatrists argued that, far from treating madness, asylums might actually produce it (a view that resurfaced in the twentieth century).

For all that, the public asylum may well have been an improvement over what had gone on before. Conditions were no doubt bad, but they were much worse in some of the private madhouses and also may well have been worse in the family. Nevertheless, doubts began to be raised about just who were being confined, and why.

Social insecurity and self-help

In 1810 the average expectation of life for males in Britain had stood at 38.7 years; by 1861 it had risen to only 40.5 years. And the crude death rate, which had been 30.7 per 1 000 as far back as 1680, had drifted down only very slowly to 24.5 per 1 000 by 1850.* It seems likely that most of what improvement in health had occurred is attributable to better nutrition and standards of living, rather than to any benefits of expanding formal health care. But why were the hospitals, workhouse infirmaries and asylums growing so rapidly? One reason was that such institutions were often

*These changes are discussed in more detail in *The Health of Nations, ibid.* Chapter 8 (U205 Book III).

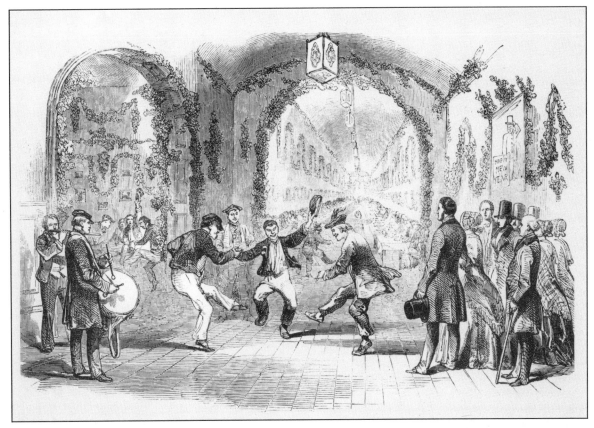

Figure 4.7 Twelfth-Night Entertainments at the Hanwell Lunatic Asylum. The Middlesex Asylum at Hanwell, with over one thousand patients in 1840, was by far the largest in the country. The reformer Dr John Conolly, on taking an appointment at Hanwell in 1839, abolished the use of mechanical restraints such as belts, wristlocks, boot hobbles and coercion-chairs, and initiated organised education for patients. The happy effects on male patients (females were segregated and had their party on New Year's Eve) are shown in this anonymous wood engraving of 1848. But Hanwell was atypical, and the visiting committee of the hospital (some of whom are shown on the right of the illustration) curbed Conolly's more ambitious reform proposals on the grounds of cost.

the last — or indeed only — refuge of people with nowhere else to go, and no means of support. Insecurity was a looming presence for much of the population, dependent on the labour market for wages that were too low to allow anything to be saved, and that could stop abruptly through accident, illness, or economic slump. Fear of finishing up in the workhouse was pervasive.

Since medieval times, craftsmen's guilds in many towns had been running *mutual benefit funds*, which gave money to members at times of sickness. In the nineteenth century these proliferated as *Friendly Societies* and medical clubs, forms of self-help that were continually encouraged by the Poor Law Commissioners. However, they were often financially unsound, spending more on social activities than medical assistance; a number had collapsed in the late eighteenth century leading to abortive proposals in Britain

to introduce state health insurance. Moreover, members who became sick or old were often debarred from benefits and finished up needing poor relief and relying on doctors for health care.

In the 1830s two societies, the Oddfellows and the Foresters, pioneered more rigorous forms of financial management, and attracted large memberships. However, the scale of medical provision from such sources was wholly inadequate to meet the demands that were placed upon them. Despite the growth in membership of the Friendly Societies (around four million by the 1870s) and the trade unions, which were particularly active in providing various sickness and other benefits, the health needs of an industrial working class could not be met. Rapid population growth, urbanisation, the factory system and economic insecurity demanded new mechanisms of social security and health care provision. Mutual self-help could be a palliative for some, but not a solution for all.

Most people relied, as they always had done, on perhaps the oldest form of mutual self-help — the family. The mutual aid provided by the family was essential to survival. Compared to the world of today, very few people lived on their own, children left home much later and they did not marry until they had both discharged their family obligations and accumulated enough resources to start a family of their own. Workers who succumbed to the hazardous industrial conditions of the early nineteenth century, through accident, illness or being laid off, depended more than anything else on the tight and, by today's standards, highly constraining network of family obligations for support and care. So too, as we have noted, did many people suffering from mental illness.

As literacy spread and book production was mechanised and made cheaper, so the influence of mass-produced health care manuals on lay care grew. Some manuals not only encouraged self-care, but gave rise to lay health movements. One such was written by a New Hampshire farmer and lay healer in America, Samuel Thompson. His *New Guide to Health* published in 1822, appeared during a time of 'therapeutic nihilism' when the activities of doctors were widely held to be of doubtful benefit. Thompson propounded remedies based on the ideas of 'Botanic Medicine', a system which made extensive use of herbs. His objective of making 'everyone his own physician' led to a major popular health movement in nineteenth-century America. The study of medicine, Thompson suggested:

> is no more necessary to mankind at large to qualify them to administer relief from pain and sickness, than to a cook in preparing food to satisfy hunger. (Cited in Starr, 1982, p.52)

Industrialisation and the introduction of mass production gave rise to another influence on lay care — proprietary medicines. The advice that accompanied the medicines often included details of the conditions for which its use was appropriate, though as the advertisement in Figure 4.8 illustrates, these claims were often extravagant.

Some now famous names established themselves during this period including Thomas Beecham, who patented his 'powders' in 1847, and Jesse Boot, who learnt his herbalism from his mother at his parent's pharmacy in Nottingham. He was to become the proprietor of the world's largest retail chemist company. Some of these proprietary medicines were harmless but ineffective, others no doubt cured or at least palliated some conditions. But a few were positively dangerous. Many patients must have become addicted to these and, according to the historian F.B. Smith, some people died from overconsumption:

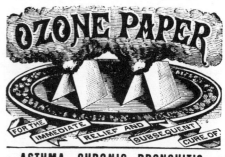

Figure 4.8 Advertisement for a proprietary medicine: 'Ozone Paper'; the immoderate claims are endorsed by a professional physician. *London Illustrated News*, 21 November, 1885.

As the foreman of a jury . . . in 1851 remarked, 'Morrison's Pills do no harm. I have a workman who takes 30 a day at a time'. The coroner capped this. He 'had an old woman at an inquest recently who used to take 300 a day'. The inquest was upon a child of five, who had had scarlet fever. Its father had bought the pills from one of Morrison's sellers . . . had fed the child about 20 pills in three days — whereupon it died. The verdict was natural death. (Smith, 1979, p.344)

Taking stock

The period up to the 1860s was in many ways a time of confusion, paradox and contradiction. Raised on *laissez-faire* foundations, poor relief had turned into a system of expanding, publicly provided, health care. Government intervention had also grown in the field of public health. The century had begun with a small number of hospitals, even with the very existence of hospitals being questioned: 'A man is made neither for trades [guilds], nor a hospital, nor for a poor-house; such a prospect is terrible', the French revolutionary Saint-Just had proclaimed, advocating their abolition and the reinstatement of the family as the sole institution for the care of the poor (cited in Foucault, 1976, p.44). By 1860 dreams of abolishing them seemed absurd; in France, as you have seen, the teaching hospital had mushroomed; in England the voluntary hospitals had grown, the workhouse infirmaries had grown, the asylums had grown. (So fast, it seemed at the time, that *The Times* was moved to comment that 'if lunacy continues to increase as at present, the insane will be in the majority, and, freeing themselves, will put the sane in asylums' — cited in Scull, 1979, p.225.)

Reform was uneven. The medical profession had begun to unite in 1858, the nurses were beginning to follow suit. Workhouse infirmary conditions had been comprehensively exposed, but concerted reforms were still in the future. Mutual self-help, in family, clubs, societies or unions, remained the main source of health care for many, at once indispensable and inadequate. And for every reform proposed, objections were made: sewage reform threatened the livelihood of human dung collectors; workhouse improvements burdened ratepayers; legislation on factory conditions caused anxiety to shareholders. These conflicts of interest were captured neatly in a conversation noted by Friedrich Engels sometime in the 1840s:

> One day I walked with one of these middle-class gentlemen into Manchester. I spoke to him about the disgraceful unhealthy slums and drew his attention to the disgusting condition of that part of town in which the factory workers lived, I declared that I had never seen so badly built a town in my life. He listened patiently and at the corner of the street, at which we parted company, he remarked: 'And yet there is a great deal of money made here. Good morning Sir'. (Engels, cited in Hobsbawm, 1962, p.218)

But as the century progressed, the growing wealth of industrial Britain was increasingly directed towards repairing the worst excesses of the Industrial Revolution, and tackling the deficiencies of health care. And amidst the propaganda and campaigning of the reformers and the counter-propaganda and blocking tactics of vested interests, developments in science and technology began to transform the nature and the effectiveness of health care.

1860–1914
Science, state and the 'sanitary idea'
With Edwin Chadwick as its chief working member, the Board of Health established under the Public Health Act of 1848 had made progress in a number of areas: indeed, the 'Age of Chadwick' has often been seen as the most exciting period in the history of British public health. It had produced some undoubted improvements. For example, there had been a long-running problem over the burial of dead bodies, with the poor often being buried in the middle of built-up areas in shallow graves, threatening disease outbreaks. In one of many similar instances, in Paisley, Renfrewshire, the discovery of one disturbed grave in 1832 had triggered such anger and fear of cholera that a demonstration by thousands ensued, ending in a riot and the smashing of the windows of the town's doctors.

Chadwick pushed for reform for many years, and in 1852 an Act gave local authorities powers to establish properly maintained cemeteries. The inequalities between poor and rich that existed even in death were reduced (see Figure 4.9).

But public health reform was caught squarely in the never-settled issues over central or local control, and private or public responsibility. Chadwick's reforming activities had aroused resentment amongst those whom he wished to make more accountable, and in 1854 he had been pressured into retirement; by 1858 the Board of Health had been wound up, and no central body existed to regulate public health.

From this point onwards, however, a number of new factors emerged. First, scientific progress in understanding

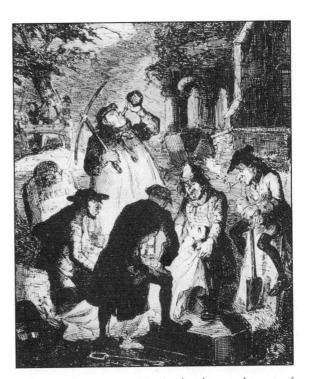

Figure 4.9 *The Resurrectionists.* Another threat to the peace of dead bodies came from the body-snatchers and grave-robbers, who met the demand from the rapidly expanding medical schools for fresh human material in anatomy instruction. Edinburgh, with the largest school, created the largest demand, and the resulting scarcity and high prices for bodies attracted the underworld. Two such operators, Burke and Hare, took the shortcut of murder, and in 1828 supplied the bodies of sixteen victims for anatomy teaching in the Surgeon's Hall. Burke was hanged, and the ensuing scandal resulted in the Anatomy Act of 1832, which allowed any unclaimed body to be claimed for dissection. The Act is still in force.

disease accelerated. Of particular importance was the development of *bacteriology*. Once infectious disease was shown to be caused by particular germs or microorganisms, rather than by miasmas, and once reliable methods of identification had been developed, not only could scientists search for methods of prevention and treatment, but also central and local authorities could engage in the routine checking of food, water and so forth. The battle against infectious disease was no longer a general assault upon 'filth' but a focused search for particular sources of infections. The precision of such routine monitoring gave authorities a powerful new weapon in their attempts to regulate and control recalcitrant towns, families, tradesmen and industrialists. With these early developments in bacteriology and the appointment of Medical Officers of Health, one of whose key tasks was to examine the quality of the water, local authorities began to take an active interest in such matters. In London, for example, from the 1860s, monthly water reports were prepared by the Registrar-General in London and the Society of Medical Officers of Health. Both the quality and quantity of water supplies had become a topic of political controversy. This enlistment of science in the cause of reform was encouraged by John Simon, who as Medical Officer to the parliamentary Privy Council had become effectively Chadwick's successor in public health administration.

Simon gathered around him a team of scientists and engineers, and their advice and assistance helped a number of towns to install sewer systems in the 1850s and 1860s. The most spectacular achievement was in London, where between 1858 and 1865 Sir Joseph Bazalgette supervised the installation of 80 miles of sewers.

Science, then, had begun to have an impact on public health. By itself, however, it was not enough: the Public Health Act of 1875, which represented the culmination of Simon's career, was essentially a move that consolidated existing powers to control the environment, and made them easier to enforce, but did not significantly extend powers to improve public health into new areas. In particular, local government was a stumbling block to effective public health reform.

One important reason for this was that, until 1867, town government rested with ratepayers, who by sanctioning town expenditure would have cut their own incomes. The narrowness of the franchise was striking: in 1861 3 per cent of Birmingham's population was eligible to vote for the town council, in Ipswich 10 per cent, in Leeds 13 per cent. But from 1867 onwards, as the franchise gradually widened, the people who stood to benefit from public health expenditure could not easily be ignored. Joseph Chamberlain in Birmingham, a leading radical liberal of the time, was one of the first to adapt to changed circumstances: in 1871–1873 his successful political campaign to become mayor of Birmingham was run on a platform of installing a city water supply and paving the streets.

Local government changed in other ways, too. Powers were given to it by central government on an increasing scale. In the 1870s it was made much easier for local authorities to take over the still predominantly private water-supply companies. In 1871 around one-third of urban authorities controlled water supplies, but by the century's end two-thirds did. The costs of creating municipal water supplies were high — London in the early 1900s spent no less than £47 million buying out private water suppliers — and so central government had to lend or give increasing amounts to local authorities. Sewage disposal required even greater sums, and between 1875 and 1900, the local authorities borrowed eight times the amount from central government to finance sewage schemes as they had borrowed in the previous twenty-five years.

Local government involvement in public health grew in scale and scope throughout the late nineteenth and early twentieth centuries: in the regulation of trades and foodstuffs, the notification of infectious disease, the provision of school medical examinations, and the control of housing standards. It was the 'golden age of local government', and as we will see shortly, it extended into hospital provision. By contrast, the direct powers of central government in health care were limited.

Without the rapid industrial expansion of the later nineteenth century, the massive investment in public health infrastructure would have been impossible. Some of this industrial wealth went straight into privately financed solutions to public health problems: a series of company new towns were built, including Port Sunlight in 1889, Bournville in 1893, and New Earswick near York in 1901. Letchworth — the first *Garden City* — in 1903, and Hampstead Garden Suburb in 1905, also attempted to integrate industry and a healthy living environment. On the other hand, powerful industrial interests ensured that many attempts at environmental reform were stillborn. As the Commission on Sewage reported at the end of the century:

> Any measure absolutely prohibiting the discharge of ... refuse into sewers might be remedying one evil at the cost of an evil still more serious in the shape of ... damage to manufacturers. (Commission on Sewage, 1898–1901, cited in Wohl, 1983, p.242)

Interests such as these prevented any serious action on river and air pollution until well into the twentieth century. The regulation of factory conditions was also a slow process: as Table 4.3 shows, the first Factory Medical Inspector was not appointed in England until 1898, and in many other European countries not until well into the twentieth century.

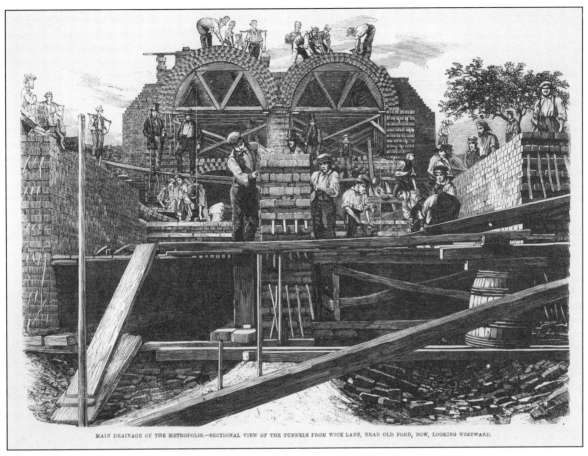

MAIN DRAINAGE OF THE METROPOLIS.—SECTIONAL VIEW OF THE TUNNELS FROM WICK LANE, NEAR OLD FORD, BOW, LOOKING WESTWARD.

Figure 4.10 6 000 men, directed by Sir Joseph Bazalgette, built London's main sewer system between 1858 and 1865: eighty miles of tunnel running north and south of the Thames with outfalls into the river at Barking and Crossness. '[T]he opening ceremonies at the southern outfall down the Thames were attended by the Prince of Wales, Prince Edward of Saxe-Weimar, the Lord Mayor, the Archbishop of Canterbury, the Archbishop of York, and 500 guests, who dined on salmon while the city's excreta gushed forth into the Thames beneath them' (Wohl, 1983, p.107).

Table 4.3 The year of appointment of the first factory medical inspectors

Country	Year
Belgium	1895
England	1898
Netherlands	1903
Baden	1906
Bavaria	1909
Italy	1912
Austria	1919
Prussia	1921
Saxony	1921
France	1942

(Source: Rosen, 1958, Table VII, p.425)

Personal health

The public health reforms of the later nineteenth century were accompanied by changes in personal health, although these are less well documented. Many changes were related to the same factors that influenced public health: the application of science, the expansion of industrial output, the extension of the franchise. Indeed public health came to be associated with domestic hygiene and cleanliness. The municipal baths and wash-houses movement, pioneered in Liverpool in the 1840s, began to mushroom, and became another object of civic pride in 'cleanliness for the masses': by the 1890s local authorities up and down the country were commissioning lavish schemes, '. . . perhaps aware of the fact that they were erecting monuments to their participation in the "sanitary idea"' (Wohl, 1983, p.75).

Washing and bathing in homes also increased: in 1853

soap tax was repealed and production increased. But the key change was in the marketing of soap: William Lever, by advertising, wrapping up and giving a brand name to his 'Sunlight' soap, increased his soap output from 3 000 tons in 1886 to 15 000 tons by 1889. His success enabled him to build Port Sunlight new town, mentioned above. How much cleaner people were is largely guesswork, as is the effect of all this activity on health: Lever's product was accompanied by a pamphlet entitled 'Sunlight Soap and How to Use It', which suggested it was something of a novelty, and even in 1894 the proportion of houses in northern English industrial towns with a fixed bath was no more than 5 per cent.

But there are fewer doubts about the impact of industry and the mass market on medicines and home cures. By the 1880s manufactured medicines were being sold in increasing amounts, and beginning to supplant more traditional home cures. An important technical innovation of the period was the compressed pill, pioneered by Burroughs Wellcome, but the essential reason for the growth of sales was probably the rise in working-class disposable income. Between 1850 and 1914 sales of manufactured medicines rose by 400 per cent (Fraser, 1981, p.139).

These developments not only affected lay health care practices in Britain, but practices throughout the British Empire and Europe. Beecham, Boot and others developed export and manufacturing divisions throughout the world, constituting the earliest multinationals catering to the pursuit of well-being through self-medication. The literature accompanying patent medicines continued to be a source of information for a lay audience until well into the twentieth century and indeed still is today.

By the end of the nineteenth century, doctors and legislators were becoming increasingly concerned about the possible harm that self-treatment could cause, and in 1909 the BMA launched a sustained attack on these 'secret remedies', their contents, and the claims made for them. Legislation was eventually passed to control the content and availability of proprietary medicines and to dampen down their more extravagant claims to effectiveness, and this probably led to fewer sudden deaths.

Hospitals in transition

Table 4.4 shows some basic statistics about the growth of hospitals in England from 1861 onwards.

As we noted earlier, by 1861 voluntary hospitals provided no more than around 18 per cent of all non-mental bed accommodation, and were increasingly specialising in acute work and refusing to deal with chronic or infectious disease cases. Publicly provided workhouse infirmaries were much more numerous, but conditions were often bad and had come under increasing criticism in the mid-nineteenth century.

The Lancet's revelations of workhouse infirmary conditions in 1866 were reinforced by the work of many others including the nursing reformers Louisa Twining and Florence Nightingale, and the Poor Law Board was forced to conduct its own inquiry resulting in a series of changes that began to transform not only Poor Law hospitals, but attitudes towards them.

The pace was set initially by the London Metropolitan Asylums Board, established by Parliament in 1867. The Board's initial attempts to establish fever and smallpox hospitals were thwarted, partly because of the opposition of residents in the areas in which they wanted to build hospitals. As a result, during the epidemics of 1869–1871, there were only 2 000 beds available in London in hastily constructed buildings, tents, workhouses and the hospital ship *Dreadnought*. In 1871, 7 912 Londoners died of smallpox out of a population of three and a quarter million. However, the Board then developed a system of hospitals along isolated parts of the River Thames and in the country around London, and the smallpox epidemic in 1884–1885 was handled, according to one commentator at least,

Table 4.4 Beds in English hospitals (excluding asylums), 1861–1938

Year	Beds in public hospitals		Beds in voluntary hospitals		Total	
	Number	Rate*	Number	Rate*	Number	Rate*
1861	50 000	2.6	11 000	0.6	61 000	3.2
1891	83 000	2.9	29 000	1.0	113 000	3.9
1911	154 000	4.3	43 000	1.2	197 000	5.5
1921	172 000	4.6	57 000	1.5	229 000	6.1
1938	176 000	4.3	87 000	2.1	263 000	6.4

* Rate = Number of beds per thousand population.
(Source: based on Abel-Smith, 1964, pp. 46, 152, 200, 353, 382–5)

'without great difficulty'. It was of greater significance, however, that although the Board's hospitals were originally intended to be used only by paupers, during the epidemics they were used by *all classes* of people. In this way the principle of *entitlement* to free treatment was established.

As the voluntary hospitals concentrated on fewer and fewer medical conditions, the responsibility of the Metropolitan Asylums Board grew. By the end of the nineteenth century it had developed into one of the largest and most effective hospital systems in the world. Manchester, Birmingham, Leeds and Liverpool rapidly followed the example of London. The deficiencies of philanthropy and self-help were being remedied by an increasingly comprehensive system of health care provided by local government. Between 1861 and 1911, as Table 4.4 shows, public hospital beds provided by municipal authorities underwent a three-fold increase.

☐ What advantages and disadvantages can you see in this system?

■ The advantages were that it gave plenty of scope for local initiative, and potentially avoided a centralised state bureaucracy. The disadvantage was that the level of provision was dependent on local factors, such as the wealth of the town. In the 1920s and 1930s, as you will see, this problem increased.

In contrast to the level of concern about workhouse infirmaries, little attention was paid to conditions in the asylums for the insane. The claims that had been made for them — that new, separate, asylums would allow *cures* to be effected — had proved to be exaggerated, and containment at low cost became the operative principle. So despite attempts to humanise care by providing a more personalised environment, the second half of the nineteenth century saw the landscape become dotted with giant asylums, 'a palace without, a workhouse within' as one commentator had put it, filled with far more people than had ever entered the older institutions. The average number of patients per asylum soared from 386 in 1860 to 1 072 by 1910, a far cry indeed from William Tuke's Retreat.

To modern eyes, however, perhaps the most striking feature of the nineteenth-century asylum was not the huge growth in the numbers of inmates — for we still classify large numbers of people as disordered — but the fact that they were so tightly confined and, perhaps relatedly, that they were overwhelmingly poor. To enter any asylum a patient had to be certified as insane, and once so certified very few ever left, except in their coffins. Although highly elaborate provision was made to prevent people being wrongly confined, certification was rarely challenged and there was little publicly expressed concern about the permanent confinement of people in separate and segregated institutions. Such attitudes did not begin to change until the twentieth century.

The rate of growth of the workhouse infirmaries and the asylums after 1860 was paralleled — indeed surpassed — by the rate of growth of the voluntary hospitals. Because the voluntary hospitals were increasingly concentrating on acute work, so they were especially affected by developments in acute care that increased the effectiveness of hospital treatment. Particularly important were the introductions of anaesthetics from the 1840s and of aseptic surgical procedures in the 1870s and 1880s.

With the introduction of safe and effective anaesthesia and asepsis, surgery became the first major area of clinical practice to be transformed by science, and surgeons were able to explore the body cavities — the chest, the abdomen and the skull — at relative leisure and with a huge reduction in mortality from infection. The impact on the hospital (as well as on the patient) was dramatic. Up to this point, for all the specialised development of the voluntary hospitals, and the creation of major teaching and research institutions around some of them, private surgery had been done in people's homes. Hospitals had been essentially for the working class. Now, however, they were also to be for the growing middle classes, and even for the upper classes. As an article in the *British Medical Journal* of 1903 pointed out:

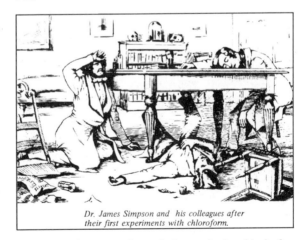

Dr. James Simpson and his colleagues after their first experiments with chloroform.

Figure 4.11 Three types of anaesthetic were developed in the first half of the nineteenth century: nitrous oxide, ether and chloroform. Dr James Simpson, professor of obstetrics at Glasgow University, discovered the anaesthetic properties of chloroform in 1847 by inhaling vapours from a tumbler in his dining-room with two colleagues. He made use of the discovery for the purpose of alleviating pain at childbirth, and within two years of his discovery it had been administered to 40 000 people in Edinburgh. Opposition, particularly theological, was widespread until Queen Victoria in 1853 accepted chloroform for the delivery of her seventh child, Prince Leopold. Sir Walter Scott is reputed to have proposed as a coat of arms for Simpson's knighthood 'a wee naked bairn' carrying the motto 'Does your mother know you're out?'

In these days of elaborate asepsis it must be recognized that almost no ordinary dwelling-house can provide the environment that is considered necessary for the achievement of the best surgical results. (Cited in Abel-Smith, 1964, p.189)

☐ What effect might this have had upon the relationships between the doctor and middle-class patient?

■ Increasingly from then on, middle-class patients went to see doctors rather than doctors going to see patients.

However, these new standards of care in the voluntary hospitals were expensive, and some were beginning to experience difficulties in meeting their running costs. In other countries, this problem had been met by the existence of pay hospitals, whereby patients were charged for services received; such hospitals were to be found by the 1870s in France, Switzerland, Spain, Germany, Austria, Norway, Sweden, Italy, the USA and Canada.

Charging patients for hospital care did begin to develop in England, although by the 1890s the proportion of hospital income raised in this way was still small: 5 per cent in London and 15 per cent elsewhere.

But the problems of the hospital services — voluntary and public — had by the end of the century become too profound to admit of piecemeal remedies. Although both types of hospital had their origins in the provision of services for the poor, they could increasingly offer effective but expensive treatments to the poor, the middling and the rich. Patients might get free care in one hospital but be charged in another, with little regard to their ability to pay: in short, the system had become a '. . . morass of anomalies' (Abel-Smith, 1964, p.217). But the Royal Commission on the Poor Laws and Relief of Distress, appointed in 1905 and presented with the opportunity of recommending fundamental changes in the whole system of public hospital care (and by implication in the voluntary hospitals also), failed to reach any unanimous conclusions, and the 'morass of anomalies' remained for the time being.

Nurses and doctors
The sheer growth in the hospital services of England — from 61 000 beds in 1861 to 197 000 by 1911 — was bound to exert a profound effect on the development of health care occupations. And as you have seen, hospital services did not simply grow, they also changed in character. So how did the occupations change? Let us consider nursing first.

On Florence Nightingale's return from the Crimea, funds donated by the public were used to establish the Nightingale Training Scheme, a corner-stone of which was the Nightingale School for Nurses, opened in association with St Thomas's Hospital, London, in 1860. The establishment of this school marked a turning-point in the development of nursing, although the reasons why this was so are open to debate. Until recently, the work of the school was taken largely on the estimation of it provided by Nightingale herself:

The whole reform in nursing both at home and abroad has consisted in this; to take all power over the nursing out of the hands of men, and put it into the hands of *one female trained head* and make her responsible for everything (regarding internal management and discipline) being carried out. (Cited in Abel-Smith, 1960, p.25)

On this account the school, despite its small output of trained nurses (forty-four per year on average), exerted immense influence because an élite cadre of highly trained nurses was emplaced in hospitals around the country and ruthlessly pushed through sweeping reforms. But recent examinations of Nightingale's correspondence have revealed that over the period 1860 to 1887, during which time the day-to-day running of the school was in the hands of Mrs Sarah Wardroper, the Superintendent, the selection, training and supervision of pupils was in fact poor:

nothing was done . . . in this period to improve technical nursing, nor the knowledge base of the nurse's work, nor to define the role of the professional nurse. The halo surrounding the name of Nightingale, and the skill . . . in dealing with incipient criticism and publicity ensured the public acceptance of a sham. (Prince, 1984, p.161)

What are we to make of this newly-acquired information? Lytton Strachey, an early and iconoclastic biographer of Nightingale, would no doubt have seized upon it as yet more ammunition to debunk his subject. In another sense, it is a salutary reminder that the historical record should not rely too heavily on people's public accounts of their own actions. But third, it might be argued that the information changes very little: the school *was* immensely influential, but the image was much more influential than the reality. What is revealed about Nightingale's skill as a campaigner, propagandist and reformer is more important than what is revealed about the St Thomas's School's actual operation.

Whatever the interpretation, the years after 1860 did see an increasing number of trained nurses as other schools became established, and standards of nursing care in the voluntary hospitals rose significantly. In the workhouse infirmaries improvements were slower. But in Liverpool, Agnes Jones, an ex-pupil of Kaiserworth and St Thomas's, pioneered nursing reform as Superintendent of the

Liverpool Workhouse Infirmary from 1865 onwards, and Louisa Twining kept the issue of workhouse infirmary nursing on the reform agenda alongside her campaign to abolish Poor Law medical relief and introduce taxation-funded public hospitals.

Towards the end of the nineteenth century nursing was growing into a huge occupation. In England and Wales the number of nurses grew from 25 000 in 1861 to 69 000 in 1901, and to nearly 154 000 by 1931. Apart from the small number of schools-trained nurses, who made up these vast numbers? Using records from a sample of English provincial hospitals, Christopher Maggs, a historian and nurse, has shown that most had, at various times, difficulty in attracting young women and had lowered the ages and standards for recruitment accordingly. Immigrants, from Ireland, Wales and Scotland, made up about 15 per cent of the recruits. As Table 4.5 shows, more than 70 per cent had previous work experience.

☐ What can you infer from Table 4.5 about the social background of nursing recruits and the social status of nursing?

■ They were mostly from a working-class background, and nursing shared a similar social status with domestic service and other manual occupations.

None the less, nursing was to move, eventually, towards the kind of licensing system achieved by doctors in 1858, though the struggle, sometimes dubbed the 'Thirty Years' War' was to prove as bitter as it had been in medicine. Florence Nightingale opposed licensing, arguing that individual assessment of the personal qualities of nurses by employers would not be bettered by an impersonal examination.

☐ Who had expressed a similar view, and when, about the licensing of doctors?

■ Plato, in the fourth century BC (see Chapter 2).

A large number of doctors, particularly in rural areas, were also opposed to the licensing of nurses as they feared that:

> Nurses might flourish their certificates in front of the patients and try to make out that they 'knew more than the doctor', while the patients might be tempted to use the nurse as a substitute for the doctor as 'you can get a nurse for very little ... while the doctor's fee is higher'. (Abel-Smith, 1960, p.75)

The case for the registration of nurses was stimulated by the establishment of a register for midwives in 1902 — a register that did not have the same constellation of interests opposed to it as that for nurses.

☐ The Midwives Act of 1902 laid down that 'no woman shall, habitually and for gain, attend women in childbirth otherwise than under the direction of a qualified medical practitioner, unless she be certified under this Act' (Chapter 17, Section 1). What strikes you about this in relation to the debate over a nurses register?

■ The Midwives Act ensured that doctors would not lose out, but would stand to gain by having more control. This was less clearly likely to be the case with nurses.

In fact, it was not until 1919 that the nurses followed the midwives: again a war had influenced profoundly the development of the occupation.

Table 4.5 Distribution of previous work experiences of recruits to nurse training, 1881–1921 (percentages)

	Manchester Royal Infirmary (1881–1921)	The London Hospital (1881–1921)	Leeds Poor Law Infirmary (1895–1921)
Nil	28	28	28
Nursing	39	26	35
Domestic service	21	29	22
Clerical and commercial	4	5	3
Clothing and textiles	1	2	5
Shop work	2	2	4
Education	5	5	2
War work and miscellaneous	1	3	1
Actual number of recruits	1 696	4 454	3 70

(Source: Maggs, 1983, Table 2.2, p.67)

The scientific developments affecting hospitals had particularly striking effects on the organisation of medical practice. During the 1860s and 1870s in Britain, the newly unified practitioners of medicine enjoyed increasing income and social status, attaining what the Prime Minister, W.E. Gladstone, described as 'equality with the other cultivated or leisured classes'. Although there were still wide disparities in doctors' incomes, there were fewer differences than before.

This greater social and economic homogeneity was, however, matched by a major intellectual and technical fragmentation. A commentator of 1888 wrote as follows:

Small portions of physic and surgery have been separated from the parent trunks and been consigned to groups of practitioners who are hence known as specialists. The eye engages the entire attention of oculists or ophthalmic surgeons; the ear of aurists or aural surgeons; the mind of lunacy doctors ... or alienists; deformities fall to the orthopaedic surgeon ... the larynx as part of 'the throat' was only a few years ago severed from the rest of the body, and the diseases were made into a speciality, owing to the necessity of using a new instrument, styled the laryngoscope, for their recognition and treatment. (Cited in Brotherston, 1971, pp.97–8)

☐   In what way was this specialisation new?
■   Traditionally, qualified doctors had dealt with a great range of conditions — only 'quacks' had specialised.

The growth of biomedical knowledge made it increasingly difficult for any single doctor to care for all conditions and categories of patient. In addition, the creation of ever larger hospitals, in which larger numbers of doctors worked, provided an opportunity for doctors to concentrate their attention in specialised areas.

In several European countries specialisation began to impede and even destroy the development of general practice, and for a while it seemed that the same might occur in England. The growth of out-patient departments in the voluntary hospitals, already noted in the earlier part of the nineteenth century, continued, causing GPs to cry 'hospital abuse' as they saw potential patients being 'poached'. Thus in 1900 a South London GP wrote of how:

a large number of working people ... pay for medical attendance at the rate of one shilling for medicine at the doctor's surgery ... If they get free advice and medicine at a hospital of course they will go there ... In bad weather they send for the GP or go to him for medicines. In fine weather they all flock to the hospitals ... [let it be] remembered that one million and a half of persons are reported to be treated at the

London Hospitals. (Cited in Brotherston, 1971, pp.102–3)

A solution to these problems was found, however, in the system of *referral*, whereby GPs obtained unique rights over the access of patients to hospitals. Whereas in other countries people, if they could afford it, could refer themselves directly to a specialist, in Britain all access to specialists was to come solely through the GP.

☐   What factors do you think led to the acceptance by specialists of a system in which access to them was controlled by GPs?
■   A number of factors appear to have contributed: generalists could select appropriate patients for the specialists; GPs were largely giving up their rights to practice in the hospitals, leaving specialists in control; and GPs were prepared to leave the care of many patients to the specialists.

Rudolf Klein, a health policy analyst, has described this as 'a demarcation agreement between two crafts, of exactly the same kind that developed between different crafts in shipbuilding and other British Industries' (Klein, 1983, p.87). Initially the split between specialist and GP was not complete. Many GPs maintained part-time posts in hospitals (a grade that still exists today in the UK). In addition, in rural areas without hospitals or specialists, GPs established their own small cottage hospitals in which they could treat their own patients, even with simple surgical operations, a trend which continued into the 1930s.

But even with the rise of the hospital, house-calls continued to be made on a great scale. These too were transformed, particularly in rural areas, by a series of technical developments in the field of *communications*:

When patients were treated at home, before the advent of the telephone, the doctor had to be summoned in person. So the costs of travel were often doubled, as two people, the physician and an emissary, had to make the trip back and forth. Furthermore, since the doctor was often out on calls, there was often no guarantee that he would be found when someone went in search of him ... Doctors were [therefore] among the earliest to buy cars. A physician who wrote to the *Journal of the American Medical Association*, which published several supplements on automobiles between 1906 and 1912, reported that with a car 'It is the same as if they had forty-eight hours instead of twenty-four'. (Starr, 1982, pp.65–75)

As with many other aspects of early twentieth-century health care and medical science, such changes were increasingly occurring first in America or Germany, and

England was once again having to adjust to the idea of importing rather than exporting the latest ideas.

Social insecurity rediscovered

With the enormous growth in all forms of health care during the nineteenth century, accompanied by rising industrial output and real incomes, it was no doubt tempting to believe at the end of the century that the worst problems of poverty and ill-health had been removed. Such beliefs were badly shaken by two events. First, extensive social survey work by Charles Booth, Seebohm Rowntree and Beatrice and Sidney Webb rediscovered the existence of widespread poverty, poor nutrition and bad housing. Once again the tradition of political arithmetic had demonstrated its persuasiveness. Second, the outbreak of the Boer War in South Africa (1899–1902) not only confirmed the existence of widespread ill-health, but also provided the lesson that such ill-health was a military liability.

According to official army statistics, of 679 703 men medically examined for enlistment between 1893 and 1902, 234 914, or just over a third, were rejected as medically unfit. Less than 10 per cent of volunteers in Manchester were considered fit enough to send abroad to fight. How, in a phrase of the time, could an 'A1 Empire be sustained by a C3 nation'? The immediate response was a government inquiry, the Interdepartmental Committee on Physical Deterioration, which called for sweeping changes. Among the recommendations initially enacted was the creation of a Schools Medical Service in 1906, and in the economic depression that followed the war, central government took other steps of direct intervention, such as in unemployment relief. A most significant step in this direction occurred in 1911, with the introduction of National Health Insurance.

During the latter part of the nineteenth century some attempts had been made to expand the existing friendly societies and clubs and to encourage the establishment of health insurance schemes. However, this was only on a voluntary basis and by 1900 a mere 13 per cent of the population were covered. Meanwhile, only half the working population were members of societies and clubs offering some form of health provision, and even this was often primitive and restricted to a few items of medical care, such as dispensary supplies of medicines. Children, the elderly and women who were not in paid employment were excluded from both insurance schemes and friendly societies.

These problems were not unique to Britain, but had been recognised throughout Europe. Following the failed revolution of 1848 in Germany, Count Otto von Bismarck, a landowner and member of the aristocracy, drew a clear lesson: 'the social insecurity of the worker is the real cause

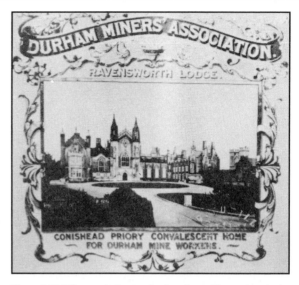

Figure 4.12 The associations and unions formed by workers in the nineteenth century often provided convalescent homes and sickness saving schemes for members. Conishead Priory was a typical example. Once owned by the Durham miners, it has since become a Buddhist college.

of their being a peril to the state'. In 1862, Bismarck became Prime Minister of the north German state of Prussia and in 1872 Chancellor of a recently formed union of north and south German states. He was therefore in a position to make use of the lessons 1848 had taught him, as the medical historian Henry Sigerist has noted:

> What Bismarck had in mind was a centralised and unified system of insurance that would protect all economically weak groups including agricultural workers from major risks by providing compensation and services. It was to be financed by contributions of employers and employees, and by government subsidies. Government charity was to become government subsidy. (Sigerist, 1943, p.376)

It was opposed by the liberals, who wanted a more *laissez-faire* system, and by the socialists, who rightly suspected that Bismarck was trying to squash their growing strength. Nevertheless, in 1883 the Sickness Insurance Act was made law, followed by an Accident Insurance Act and a Pension and Invalidity Insurance Act. The idea of the *welfare state* had been born.

Compulsory sickness insurance schemes spread to Austria in 1888, Hungary in 1892, Norway in 1909, and Russia in 1912, while other European governments such as Sweden and Denmark, began to give extensive state aid to the voluntary insurance societies. Britain was one of the later countries to adopt the system. In 1908, old age pensions were introduced (except for those who were held

THE DAWN OF HOPE.

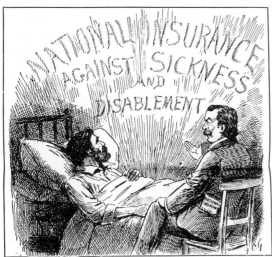

Mr. LLOYD GEORGE'S National Health Insurance Bill provides for the insurance of the Worker in case of Sickness.

Support the Liberal Government
in their policy of
SOCIAL REFORM.

Figure 4.13 Lloyd George poster of 1911. The Act of 1911 established for the first time in Britain the concept of benefits as a right based on records of contributions.

to have been work-shy and improvident) and in 1911 the then Chancellor of the Exchequer, Lloyd George, introduced his scheme for National Health Insurance. Like Bismarck, Lloyd George was well aware of the growing parliamentary representation of the socialists and the electoral power which the extension of the franchise in 1885 had given to working-class men. Although he had paid close attention to Bismarck's scheme, he failed to avoid repeating the German system's weaknesses. Cash benefits for sickness, accident and disability were not centralised under the scheme, but continued to be distributed through existing insurance companies and societies. They were left with considerable discretion in deciding what cash and medical benefits to provide, and so there were no uniform rights. What the National Health Insurance Act did guarantee, however, was the provision of medical services from general practitioners. The Act gave GPs a list, or 'panel', of insured workers, for each of whom the GP received a 'capitation' fee. Although panel patients received free treatment, their dependants did not. The latter either had to pay health care costs privately or join their own 'insurance clubs'. In addition to 'panel' patients, some GPs

were able to build up a lucrative practice seeing wealthy patients privately. The hard fight GPs mounted to retain this privilege left Lloyd George of the opinion that doctors were 'both unreasonable and unruly', and the retention of private medical practice alongside the 'panel work' of insurance doctors meant that in industrial areas of the north, and in inner city areas, GPs were quite poorly paid and often each had lists of between four and five thousand panel patients or dependants. In wealthier areas, however, such as West London and the home counties, GPs could have lists of fewer than one thousand — mainly private patients, and still make a very comfortable living.

The actions of central government in the aftermath of the Boer War were significant for a number of reasons, but perhaps above all they:

> ... marked the end of the growing preponderance of the local authorities in public service. As the new schemes had immense potentialities of expansion (which were just beginning to show themselves by 1914) the trend towards centralisation was bound to become more and more marked. (Ashton, 1960, pp.228–9)

1914–1939

As we have seen, the opening years of the twentieth century saw a whole series of changes in British health care, and indeed in British society.

Why, then, punctuate this section at the year 1914, the beginning of the First World War? There are two main reasons.

First, the First World War was the first full-scale conflict between industrial countries using industrial methods of mechanised warfare; in consequence the scale of human death and injury was immense and had a profound direct impact on health care. Between 1914 and 1918, 8 million people were killed in the war; 745 000 of these were from Britain, representing 9 per cent of all men aged 20 to 45. A further 1.7 million men from Britain were wounded, 1.2 million of them sufficiently badly to qualify thereafter for disablement benefit. A host of previously unknown or rare injuries and illnesses, such as gas-damaged lungs and eyes, and shell-shock, became prevalent, forcing changes in methods of care.

Moreover, the fighting was close at hand, and railways and steamships brought it even closer: Ypres, for example, was a mere 30 miles from Dunkirk, and on the day after the first battle there in November 1914, no fewer than fifty-seven trainloads of wounded soldiers arrived in London. The government was obliged, therefore, to intervene in the whole system of medical provision and health care.

But, second, the First World War marked a period of political, social and intellectual change that would subsequently exert many new influences on health care. For example, women were mobilised in large numbers into munitions and other industrial work; 120 000 women were deployed as additional wartime nurses in Voluntary Aid Detachments (VADs), and whereas in 1913 hunger-striking women seeking emancipation and the vote were being force-fed in prison, in 1918 the franchise was extended with little serious opposition to all women over 30 years of age. Finally, whereas the pre-war period had seen state intervention and concern focus on child and maternal welfare, the war forced along the idea that the state must also intervene in issues affecting the health of all adult citizens. These changes were manifested in a series of proposals for the reform of health care, and inquiries into existing services and conditions. Many of the organisational changes required to implement these ideas were delayed until the aftermath of the Second World War, as you will see in the next chapter, but it was in the inter-war period that the ideas themselves took hold. This is reflected particularly well in developments in public health.

Public health

The main concerns of public health during the nineteenth century have already been described.

☐ How would you summarise the focus of attention of public health in the nineteenth century, particularly in the period from Chadwick to the 1875 Public Health Act?

■ Essentially the focus was on the environmental circumstances in which ill-health prospered: water, sewage, sanitation and ventilation had to be improved.

Although nineteenth-century public health measures had focused almost entirely on the environment, an interest in *personal* health had become widespread amongst the middle and upper classes.

Thus the 1860s had seen a huge emphasis on the importance of physical exercise for health; an emphasis reflected in the nation-wide development of gymnasia and athletics festivals as well as in the creation of new types of organised sports (many of which date from this period) and the beginnings of compulsory games in schools. Alongside this emphasis on exercise there was a growing emphasis on systematic popular education concerning the new scientific knowledge of health and disease. In 1867, in his inaugural address as Rector of Aberdeen University, the philosopher and economist John Stuart Mill urged that physiology be made a part of everyone's programme of study (Haley, 1978, p.17). Such trends had not reached the working classes, however, and personal health was still left primarily to the individual and to voluntary organisations.

But towards the end of the nineteenth century the 'sanitary idea' was beginning to give way to, first, the idea

that public health could be further advanced by turning attention to individuals and to personal health measures in all social classes, and second, the related idea that this could only be done through the creation of systematic procedures for surveying, monitoring and keeping track of individuals and their state of health. This was a trend that accelerated in the years up to 1939.

The move from environmental to personal health measures was of course far more than a simple, technical re-orientation. It involved a principle: of communal responsibility for *individuals* (particularly children and pregnant women) as well as the environment in which they lived.

But once the principle had been conceded over maternal and child welfare, it became easier to extend it to other issues. Tuberculosis and venereal disease came next.

The National Tuberculosis Association, founded in 1898, had run an effective propaganda campaign on the disease and the need for something more than environmental improvements to tackle it. Part of the problem was that the disease is of indefinite length, and any acceptance of communal responsibility for persons affected would therefore be open-ended. By 1912 a requirement had been laid down that local Medical Officers of Health be notified of the disease, but in 1921 this system was still far from perfect: in Barnsley that year, 87 per cent of tuberculosis deaths occurred among people of whom the MOH had been notified not at all or very late.

Gradually the systems of recording and monitoring, of surveillance and of notification spread, until by 1936 it was compulsory to maintain registers not only of sufferers, but of all contacts also, and to maintain them for four years after each notification. The campaign also involved direct assistance from the Exchequer for the provision of sanatoria, which expanded from 5 500 beds in 1911 to almost 29 000 beds by 1934. It also became a movement to provide special houses for tuberculous patients after their discharge from sanatoria, and emphasis was laid increasingly on treating *all* patients irrespective of financial status. The direction of public health policy was therefore more and more towards universal provision of care for individual tuberculous patients.

Parallel developments can be observed in the treatment of venereal diseases. These had been a source of continual anxiety during the First World War, with approximately 25 per cent of soldiers in the armies of Europe incapacitated by venereal disease at some stage in the conflict. The British Army had tried a system of deterrence, charging soldiers who contracted venereal disease for their own treatment and stopping their pay: some soldiers were leaving hospital in debt. But it was also a civilian problem, and in 1916 and 1917 legislation was enacted empowering local health authorities to provide diagnosis and treatment (the cost

HEALTHABET

A for Ambition to thrive and be wealthy.
B for the Baby that's happy if healthy.
C for the Children taught to be clean.
D for the Dirt that brings illness unseen.
E for Enjoyment that cleanliness brings.
F for the Fight against all filthy things.
G for the Germs you should wash right away.
H for the Health you improve every day.
I for Infection wherever you go.
J for the Jollity healthy folk know.
K for the Knowledge that dirt is wrong.
L for Life that is healthy and long.
M for Microbes that swarm everywhere.
N for Neglect that gives them a lair.
O for Often—to wash often is right.
P for Pride in your home clean and bright.
Q for the Quick way to banish all ill.
R for the Right way—clean with a will.
S for Sickness, in dirty homes rife.
T for Teaching a healthier life.
U for Ugliness dirt spreads about.
V for the Vigour that cleans it all out.
W for Washing—that watchword of purity.
X for eXcellent health and security.
Y for Youth—they're the Nation to-morrow.
Z for the Zeal that makes health banish sorrow.

Published by HEALTH & CLEANLINESS COUNCIL, 5, Tavistock Sq., London. W.C.1.

Figure 4.14 A 'Healthabet' card issued by the Health and Cleanliness Council in the inter-war period. The motto of the Council: 'Where there's dirt there's danger'.

aided by the Exchequer), and to promote propaganda and educational measures. The National Council for Combating Venereal Disease became the main body for such measures, holding meetings (24 000 by 1931, attended by five million people), encouraging biology lessons in schools, and distributing books, pamphlets and films: 'Damaged Lives', a typical offering, was seen by four million people in 327 towns (Weeks, 1981, p.211).

Health education, therefore, was emerging around this time as a key component of public health. The state would accept responsibility for individual health matters, but individuals had also to accept responsibility for their own health. Education to promote health was particularly marked in the work of the Medical Officers of Health, and

it was their Society in 1927 that brought into being the Central Council for Health Education (later to become the Health Education Council).

The movement towards education in health also manifested itself in the development of public health nursing. Beginning in 1862 'when the Ladies Section of the Manchester and Salford Sanitary Association undertook to spread health information among the poor of the community' (Rosen, 1958, p.376), visiting nurses spread rapidly to other areas, promoting in particular the care and welfare of young children at home.

☐ What early twentieth-century events would have been likely to encourage the spread of health visitors?
■ The child and maternal welfare movement, mentioned earlier, and its accompanying legislation.

By 1918 the number of health visitors had reached 3 000, and by 1919 uniform training requirements had been laid down.

The view underlying the creation of health visitors was that individuals could improve their own state of health by changing aspects of their lifestyle, in particular, standards of personal hygiene. This is evident in such activities as the 'Health Weeks' held in the industrial city of Salford during the 1920s. Their aim, as the extract from the local newspaper in Figure 4.15 illustrates, was to create a 'public health conscience'.

☐ How, according to the campaign, were 'men and women' expected to prevent disease?
■ (i) Through knowledge and observance of the 'rules governing health'.
(ii) Through proper use of services such as ante-natal services and welfare centres.
(iii) Through control of 'bad' habits such as spitting (held to pass on TB).
☐ Which members of the family did the speakers consider were responsible for promoting health?
■ Women. As Dr Brade-Birks noted in her lecture: 'Improved conditions could only be created by greater interest on the part of women'.

Did this great wave of teaching, education, propaganda and campaigning about health have an effect? On this question we must note that the more formal aspects of health education in the 1920s and 1930s became closely connected to a series of changes in fashion and pastimes, changes which now also affected the working classes: swimming, bicycling, youth hostelling, camping, walking, all acquired an advertising value through their associations with hygiene, health and beauty. Reflecting on the changes he had witnessed between 1921 and 1931 as a Medical Officer of Health on the south coast of England, J.M. Mackintosh noted that:

SALFORD HEALTH WEEK

Large audiences at lectures

The health Committee, of which Alderman E. Desquesnes is chairman, with commendable enterprise arranged a 'health week', which began on Monday and concludes on Sunday, with a view to bringing prominently to the notice of the public these important questions and with a view to securing their co-operation.

A series of lectures

The first meeting of the series, that for women only, held in Broughton Town Hall on Monday, awarded a typical indication of the interest now being taken in health problems by women.

Mrs. E. Cuddeford, J.P., presided, Dr. Brade-Birks, in the course of her lecture, dwelt on the importance of 'health week' to the women of Salford, and stressed the special necessity that women in the home should have regard to the rules governing health. Improved conditions could only be created by greater interest on the part of women. She alluded to the infant mortality rate and said that if only a proper use was made by women of the ante-natal clinics a great deal of the high infant mortality would be reduced. The lecturer urged greater use of the welfare centres after the birth of the child.

A public health conscience

Mr. Partington, in his address, said that the 'health week' effort was not only confined to Salford, for during this week Salford was taking part in what was a national institution. The object they had in view was to create by means of lectures and cinematograph films what might be termed a public health conscience. In other words, they were trying to get men and women to realise that the prevention of disease was better than the curing of it and that the prevention was in the hands not of the medical men and women but the public themselves. He mentioned the objectionable habit of spitting in public vehicles, and said that legislation was impossible. The people had to be taught the danger of such habits. Referring to mortality among children, he said that in 1933 there were 700,000 babies born in this country. Out of these 52,582 died before attaining one year of age. Of these 32,000 died before reaching the age of three months, while 5,000 mothers lost their lives in giving them birth.

Alderman E. Desquesnes, chairman of the Health Committee, said that the reason for holding a 'health week' could be summed up in the words 'prevention is better than cure'. There was a point when one health authority could do little without the cooperation of the people themselves. The lectures which had been arranged were to show the public how they might help themselves.

(*The Reporter*,
November 21, 1925)

Figure 4.15 Salford Health Week.

In my early days in Dorset it was a commonplace to find a child sewn up for the winter; and not a few young men and women whom I had to examine as tuberculosis officer showed the most remarkable tidemarks of filth just below the line of their outer clothing', but that in 1931, when 'the fashion of the day dictates that a young woman shall wear short skirts and short hair; that she shall appear in the open air and on the seashore in light and attractive clothing, then she must be clean. There is no alternative. Then the young men who parade on the beach will learn that they are unacceptable unless they also are (in the soap-and-water sense) fresh and clean. (Mackintosh, 1953, p.108)

Hospitals, occupations and the Ministry

If the welter of Commissions, Boards, Departments, Offices, Officers, Authorities, Councils, Governors, Guardians and Inspectors involved in the running of health and medical services in the early twentieth century seems confusing to the modern observer, some comfort may be gained by the knowledge that many contemporary observers were equally bewildered. In fact, the whole machinery of government and administration proved grossly inadequate to the task of coordinating a war effort, and the organisation of the health services was merely symptomatic of a more general chaos. 'It was', noted A.J.P. Taylor, 'a last experiment in running a great war on the principles of *laissez-faire*' (1965, p.34), the only clear exception being Lloyd George's Ministry of Munitions, which by the end of the war was directing the labour of three million workers, and had demonstrated the possibilities of decisive government intervention by, for example, requisitioning 1.5 million sandbags on one Saturday afternoon in Liverpool! During the war, a series of committees was formed to consider the whole matter of post-war reconstruction, and one of the proposals to emerge from the Ministry of Reconstruction under which these committees were gathered was the creation of a Ministry of Health. Action on this proposal was stimulated by the influenza epidemic of 1918–1919, which caused at least 10 000 deaths in London alone.

Set up in the spring of 1919, the Ministry of Health was

an attempt at regrouping. It brought together responsibilities for the National Insurance scheme, under which the health insurance system was growing; all the Poor Law hospitals and the public health services of local government; the health services which had grown up in the Board of Education during the child and maternal welfare movement; and other miscellaneous responsibilities for health matters. It did not, however, group all the health services together, and in particular the hospitals remained uncoordinated. While the Ministry of Health now had responsibility for the Poor Law hospitals, the local authorities retained control of the old county asylums and municipal hospitals, plus the sanatoria and other institutions they had built, and finally the voluntary hospitals were left with their independence. The consequences of this lack of coordination, and what might be done, became a recurring theme of the period.

An early act of Dr Christopher Addison, the first Minister of Health, was to appoint in late 1919 a council 'to consider and make recommendations as to the scheme or schemes requisite for the systematised provision of such forms of medical and allied services as should, in the opinion of the Council, be available for the inhabitants of a given area'. This remit was an open opportunity for the council to start from scratch in designing a health service, and drawing on his experience of army medical organisation the chairman, Major-General Bertrand Dawson seized his chance. The report, published in 1920, has been variously described as 'a guiding star in many parts of the world', 'the parent of all regional schemes of health', and 'one of the founding documents of the National Health Service' (Watkin, 1975, p.111).

The report envisaged the bringing together of all preventive and curative services, and all communal and individual medicine, in a universal system of provision based on a nation-wide network of *health centres*. What were these health centres? The very term seemed a novelty to many at the time, but in fact they had made an appearance in the USA between 1910 and 1915. Their essence was the coordination of a range of services in a single centre serving a defined population. In 1910 in Pittsburgh one of the first health centres drew on the department store model by bringing a number of different clinics or 'health departments' under one roof. By 1919 there were at least 76 health centres in the USA, by 1930 at least 1 511.

In the Dawson scheme, the basic coordination of all preventive and curative services in a neighbourhood was to be conducted through *primary* health centres, staffed by general practitioners, nurses, midwives, dentists and visiting consultants, and equipped with a small number of beds, plus laboratories, baths and a range of recreational and keep-fit facilities. These would in turn be linked to a smaller number of more specialised *secondary* health centres, with a larger number of beds staffed mainly by consultants, to whom more difficult cases could be referred. Finally, the secondary health centres would be linked to a small number of regional teaching hospitals. The advantages of the system, it was argued, would be twofold: it would place all the best available methods of prevention and cure at the disposal of all citizens, and it would improve upon the existing best methods by fostering an intellectual traffic between doctors.

☐ Comparing the proposals for primary and secondary health centres with the health centres now in existence, what differences strike you?

■ Perhaps the most obvious difference is that the Dawson health centres contained in-patients' accommodation: in fact, they were in some respects hospitals. Modern health centres do not have in-patient facilities. Another difference is that the emphasis on recreation, keep-fit and 'physical culture' in the Dawson proposals finds no place in modern health centres; sports centres have appeared in their stead.

The report was initially well-received, but within months had been shelved. While the health centre concept proceeded apace in the United States, and in Russia polyclinics were well established as the basic unit of health care organisation, in Britain, only some ten health centres had been erected by 1939, and only one, at Peckham in London, had attracted any great attention.

The reasons for the rapid abandonment of the proposals can be found largely in the wider circumstances of the period: the government was pre-occupied with political and economic turmoil in Europe, with widespread labour unrest, and with the sudden collapse of the post-war boom. The last had particular consequences for the hospitals, to which we can now turn.

The voluntary hospitals during the war had expanded substantially, and had come to rely on public authorities for around 25 per cent of their income. But the 75 per cent coming from other sources included an element of fixed income from bequests and donations, and in a time of rapid inflation the real value of this income was falling; more important, the hospitals were bigger and more expensive to run than ever. In consequence, increasing numbers of voluntary hospitals broke with precedent and began to charge patients: between 1920 and 1921, for example, the proportion of income that the London teaching hospitals obtained from patient charges jumped from 10 per cent to 25 per cent. Thereafter, the charging of patients was placed on a different footing: hospitals increasingly formed contributory schemes, whereby pre-payments were made in return for access to services. In Sheffield, for example, the four voluntary hospitals by 1929 were raising 60 per cent of their income through a scheme in which contributions of a penny in the pound were deducted at source by employers, who added one third to the employee contributions and forwarded the total to the hospitals. In return employees were entitled to hospital care (Abel-Smith, 1964, p.327). Another of these schemes started at the time was the British Provident Association, later to become the country's largest private health insurance company.

These developments were not universally welcomed. The Labour Party by 1922 was drawing attention to the likelihood that patients too poor to meet the contributory payments, that is, patients for whom these hospitals had originally been founded, would be increasingly neglected and excluded. The BMA, also, was worried at the idea of the contributory associations or hospitals receiving payments for the services the doctors were providing, while the doctors remained unpaid. They campaigned vigorously for change, negotiated an agreement and by 1924 the payment of medical staff by the hospitals was spreading.

The GPs were also worried, fearing that the referral system they had negotiated at the turn of the century would be short-circuited by patients being directly admitted to hospitals as contributors entitled to access. Although their worst fears were not confirmed, many GPs resorted to establishing cottage hospitals, the number of which expanded rapidly, from fewer than 200 at the turn of the century to over 600 by 1935.

Two points may be drawn from the growth of the GP cottage hospitals. First, they ensured that general practitioners continued to be involved in surgery on a substantial scale: in 1938–1939 it was estimated that 2.5 million surgical operations were performed by GPs — an average of three per doctor per week (Brotherston, 1971, p.100). Surgery as a preserve of specialist surgeons is a recent phenomenon. Second, the growth of these hospitals was indicative of a lack of planning in the voluntary sector as a whole.

Because of the dependence on donations, bequests and wills, hospitals were usually small and often in a place deemed appropriate by the benefactor but not appropriate to the distribution of the population. In London, some attempt to tackle this problem was made by the King Edward's Hospital Fund, which in the inter-war period acted increasingly as a 'clearing-house' for donations and bequests, directing them in accordance with some overall conception of a rational system. Elsewhere planning proved elusive.

It is also worth stressing that in some respects some voluntary hospitals were run on highly traditional, even amateurish, lines. The autobiography of a Scottish surgeon, George Mair, recalls his great surprise at coming to work at a small voluntary hospital in Warwickshire at the beginning of 1939 (Mair, 1974): the Board which ran the hospital could still behave in the manner of the eighteenth-century subscribers — Mair was expected to pass on confidential information about the illnesses of patients who were employees, servants or merely known to board-members. A similar lack of anonymity applied to the operating theatre — the chief surgeon invited female admirers to watch him perform. And technical standards were very low — newly-appointed junior surgeons were expected to conduct a range of operations of which they had no previous experience.

Moreover, in the much more prestigious teaching hospitals, technical standards had begun to fall behind those of the USA. The best American medical schools, such as John Hopkins at Baltimore, had made research an essential component of medical careers and after the First World War, American medicine took a commanding lead over that of Europe, as science began to be applied to medicine on an almost industrial scale. By contrast, some European teaching hospitals were now slumbering quietly on the accumulated honours of the past. In France, the ideas of the medically-trained anatomists and pathologists who had created many of the triumphs of early nineteenth-century medicine still dominated the medical schools, which excluded from the curriculum natural science subjects such as physiology and biochemistry. And this despite the fact that so much of medical progress from the late nineteenth century onwards was based on these subjects which had first been developed by French scientists such as Bernard and Pasteur. Some of the same hostility towards the basic sciences could also be found in Britain. Many London teaching hospitals, for example, were reluctant to embrace the American emphasis upon research, preferring instead, as their critics put it, to concentrate upon the training of gentlemen who would be best fitted to work in the quiet of small cathedral towns. One doctor described the reaction when, in 1938, he decided to leave London and accept a pure research chair in Oxford:

> so ... I became a professor, much to the surprise, indeed consternation of relatives, friends and colleagues, who were disturbed that I should turn aside from the heights of consultant practice. (Witts, 1971, p.319)

But while at least the financial environment of the voluntary hospitals was transformed for the better by the new schemes and the era of falling prices that began in 1921, the financial environment of the public hospitals became worse. As public expenditure was squeezed, the whole tenor of debate in the Ministry of Health became one of economy. Consequently there was no growth to match that in the voluntary sector.

The Poor Law hospitals administered under the Ministry still carried associations of pauperism and deterrence, and in 1929 the penultimate step towards disassociating hospital care from the Poor Law was taken when the Local Government Act transferred the Poor Law hospitals to local authorities. In some areas the local authorities were in a position to take this opportunity to develop an integrated public hospital service, but in other areas there were obstacles: either the Poor Law buildings were simply inappropriate, or the local authority's administrative area was inappropriate, or the Poor Law Guardians changed hats but perpetuated their traditions, or simply the local authorities lacked money in depression years to develop their services.

Some definite improvements did occur, however; not least in the asylums. There, attempts had been made to separate different categories of inmates: the 'demented' from the 'lunatic', the 'lunatic' from the 'idiot', and so forth. The first attempt to define such categories in law was the passing of the Mental Deficiency Act in 1914. As with many other such Acts, its initial implementation was slow. But prompted perhaps by the experience of very large numbers of shell-shocked soldiers returning from the First World War, a new interest began to be taken in the way asylums were actually run. This is revealed in the following extract from an official report in the 1930s:

> Only advanced dementia would reconcile the average woman to the type of garment still worn in some hospitals ... A good hair cut and shampoo have a real tonic value ... the woman who is content to wear her hair untrimmed and a frock like a sack certainly is not normal. (Cited in Jones, 1972, p.257)

By the 1930s most asylums had made at least some attempt to introduce recreational facilities, show films, and develop games and a few, influenced by the Dutch, had started to introduce occupational therapy — the idea that the insane might benefit from work had returned. The rigid sexual segregation of the Victorian asylum was also slowly abolished.

Wards began to be unlocked too. Where once most patients were locked into day or night-rooms most of the time, now some were allowed to walk around the hospital, to enter the grounds, even to go beyond the walls on 'outside' or 'weekend parole'. And in line with all this, the names changed too. The 1929 Local Government Act abolished the terms 'pauper' and 'Poor Law' and the Mental Treatment Act of the succeeding year turned 'asylum' into 'mental hospital' and 'lunatic' into 'patient' or 'person of unsound mind'.

A third major change lay in the relationship between the patients in the asylum and the outside world. Although out-patient services had been developed on an enormous scale in nineteenth-century voluntary hospitals, there had been no equivalent development in the asylum. However, in 1923 the Maudsley Hospital in London was opened to the public, funded mostly by the London County Council, and offering out-patient services for the first time. At the same time the LCC was also developing an extensive after-care service, which tried to cater for the problems that mental patients faced on their discharge. The notions that some patients might recover and that not every patient needed to be locked away were gaining ground rapidly. There was a return to the optimism of the late eighteenth and early nineteenth centuries.

By the 1930s, therefore, the hospitals of Britain had developed into two systems which in many respects ran in parallel, each offering some services not provided by the other, each with limitations that owed something to the fact that a parallel system existed, for attempts at voluntary liaison and cooperation were generally unsuccessful.

What effect did hospital development have on health care occupations? We have already touched on the doctors. Despite the steady growth in hospitals and in medical services, the growth in the number of doctors was modest: in 1911 there were some 36 000 doctors and dentists, in 1921 38 000 and in 1931 46 000. The proportion of these who were women was less than 10 per cent. The growth in the number of nurses, however, was more striking.

The inter-war period for nursing began with the Nurses Registration Act of 1919, which represented the first legal attempt to define nursing. The introduction of licensing was not without its problems. The General Nursing Council, which had been handed responsibility for defining the criteria for registration, was pursuing a policy of exclusion, and was particularly concerned that the large number of women demobilising from the wartime Voluntary Aid Detachments should not be allowed to 'pose as nurses'. Many practising nurses did not meet the requirements for registration, and yet still regarded themselves or were regarded by others as *bona fide* nurses. Their discontent was exacerbated when the dentists, who obtained approval for their own register in 1921, simply admitted everyone who was at that time practising as a dentist, regardless of their training.

The state had become a substantial employer of nurses and had no wish to grant registered nurses a complete stranglehold when it was possible to keep the ranks of nursing more open, and therefore the costs down. Moreover, in the Ministry of Health it had a newly acquired means of expressing its interests. In 1922 the Ministry intervened: if the General Nursing Council did not alter its ways, threatened Minister for Health Sir Alfred Mond, 'many of the nurses would be dead and buried before they got on the register' (cited in Abel-Smith, 1960, p.104).

Registration accelerated after this intervention, but the issue of who should and who should not be on the register

Table 4.6 Membership of the National Health Insurance Scheme 1918–1936

	1918		1936	
	Number of societies	Number of members	Number of societies	Number of members
Friendly Societies	9 766	7 653 000	6 386	8 143 000
Industrial Societies	36	6 930 000	37	8 464 000
Trade Union and other Societies	360	1 668 000	184	1 561 000
Total	10 162	16 251 000	6 607	18 168 000
Percentage of total population covered		39		40

(Source: derived from Carpenter, 1984, Table 1, p.82)

was not resolved; moreover, it was an issue in which the Ministry of Health continued to play an important role. During the 1920s and 1930s, as the hospitals continued to expand, so too increasing efforts were made to recruit more trained nurses, and the 'nursing shortage' came to dominate the period. While the nursing leadership tried to defend the position that registered nurses should be employed in preference to the unregistered, the Ministry was reluctant to support this policy, not least on grounds of cost. Unregistered nurses were hired in increasing numbers, and trade union militancy spread amongst them for better conditions and pay.

On the eve of the Second World War the Athlone Committee, appointed by the Minister of Health, recommended that a second level of nurse be trained and recognised — the enrolled nurse — marking another step towards the emergence of a formal hierarchy of nursing grades. (It is instructive to note against this history the decision of the Secretary of State for Social Services in 1984 to overrule the Royal College of Nursing in their attempt to exclude unqualified nurses from the newly-formed Pay Review Body.)

Finally, let us look briefly at the state of the National Health Insurance scheme in the inter-war years. During the First World War the societies participating in the scheme

had experienced good times: low pay-outs of benefits and high incomes. However, as recession turned to depression in the 1920s, the scheme experienced increasing difficulties. As Table 4.6 shows, the number of friendly societies fell sharply between 1918 and 1936 as almost one-third went out of existence. The large industrial societies, often indirectly controlled by profit-making industrial insurance companies, meanwhile grew in strength, a trend confirming that 'the Liberals' vision of an insurance scheme run by the insured themselves was only a pious hope' (Carpenter, 1984, p.81). And underlying these developments was the stubborn persistence of mass unemployment, which made it impossible for many to maintain contributions. In consequence, by 1934 four and a half million members were in danger of having sickness benefits reduced, and three-quarters of a million faced the prospect of losing all benefits. Central government provided cash injections to stave off crisis, but the system proved unable to do much more than survive, and by the late 1930s the proportion of the population covered was almost exactly the same as it had been twenty years earlier. With the return of war in 1939, the workings of the National Health Insurance Scheme, like so much else, would be placed under the closest scrutiny.

Objectives for Chapter 4

When you have finished studying this chapter, you should be able to:

4.1 Outline the initial health problems which were a consequence of the Industrial Revolution, and some of the different solutions offered.

4.2 Discuss how the debate concerning individual or state responsibility for people's health in Britain resulted in a more centralised, state control of public health measures, the regulation of health occupations and the provision of institutions.

4.3 Describe the changing emphases of the British public health movement in the period covered by the chapter.

4.4 Provide examples of the impact of scientific and technological change on health care in the nineteenth and early twentieth centuries.

4.5 Outline the trend in Europe towards social security systems providing health insurance, and the way this trend was manifested in Britain.

4.6 Discuss the way in which the conditions and work of voluntary, Poor Law and asylum hospitals changed in the period covered by the chapter.

Questions for Chapter 4

1 (*Objective 4.1*) In 1848, Rudolf Virchow founded a new journal called *Medical Reform*, with the slogan:

Medicine is a social science and politics nothing but medicine on a grand scale.

Four decades later, Sir John Simon noted that 'even with the high civilisation of this country, and with its unequalled system of poor law relief, *privation* still exists as a cause of premature death' (cited in Jones, 1979, p.14).

What view of the underlying cause of death and disease did both writers hold? What changes were necessary to bring about an improvement in health?

2 (*Objective 4.2*) In the early nineteenth century, medicine was only a part-time economic activity for many practitioners. The 1847 Medical Directories advertise a range of general practitioners:

J. BREACH Gen: Pract: Ashton-up-Thorpe MRCS 1837 LSA 1837, surgeon to the Wallingford Union.

Edw. STEPHENS Gen: Pract: Bridge St. Manchester. LSA 1825: M.D. Leyden: FRCS (by examination) 1845: MD Berlin 1828. Covis: Surgeon Lying-In Hospital. Lecturer in Anatomy, Physiology, Morbid Anatomy and Pathology: Member: Manchester Literary and Philosophical Society: Many Publications.

I. POPJAY: Surgeon Apothecary and Midwife etc.; draws teeth and bleeds on lowest terms. Confectionery, Tobacco, Snuff, Tea, Coffee, Sugar, and all sorts of perfumery sold here. NB New laid eggs every morning by Mrs. Popjay.

To what extent was the state involved in the provision of personal health care in 1847? How did state involvement change in the latter half of the nineteenth century?

3 (*Objective 4.3*) In the 1920s and 1930s there appears to have been a good deal of emphasis placed on health education. How novel was this phenomenon, and how does it square with broader public health developments?

4 (*Objective 4.4*) Lay care and personal health, like other aspects of health care, were profoundly affected by scientific and technological changes. What aspects of this can you think of in the late nineteenth century?

5 (*Objective 4.5*) Bismarck's health insurance scheme allowed many different insurance funds, societies and clubs to continue their independent existence under the 'umbrella' of the national scheme. How did this compare with Lloyd George's scheme?

6 (*Objective 4.6*) How would you assess the relative importance of the voluntary and Poor Law hospital systems in terms of (i) status (ii) size, and (iii) standards of care in the early twentieth century?

5

War, welfare and the present

Basic issues can be dodged in a short war but not in a long one like that in which we are engaged. Social Security is the major domestic war aim of every country that has not yet solved the problem. (Sigerist, 1943, p.365)

Writing this during the Second World War, Henry Sigerist was drawing on his awareness as a medical historian of the profound influence that wars have so often seemed to exert on the development of health care and medicine. The influence of war has taken many different forms. Medical practice, for example, has often been affected by the consequences of fighting, from the high proportion of their time Greek physicians devoted to tending javelin wounds and fractures to the transformation of nursing at the military hospital in Scutari. But the Second World War, where this chapter begins, influenced health care in Britain in a more far-reaching way than any other. We can see why this should have been so by following the thoughts of Richard Titmuss, the official historian of British social policy during the war. Titmuss noted that as each war in recent history had exceeded the previous one in intensity, so concern had grown on the part of the state about the quantity and quality of the population. There were four clearly defined stages in this process. First, there was a concern that a sufficient *quantity* of men was available to form armies. Second, there was a concern to apply standards of *quality* — of physical and psychological fitness — to recruits, and to make basic health care provisions for those recruited. Third, government concern broadened to include the quality not only of existing recruits, but also of the next generation of recruits, and therefore to include that part of the population from which they were drawn. In Britain this stage was reached with the Boer War of 1899–1902, when the Inspector-General of Recruiting anxiously drew attention to 'the gradual deterioration of the physique of the working class from whom the bulk of recruits must always be drawn' (cited in

Titmuss, 1976, p.80). There followed, as the previous chapter showed, a Schools Medical Service, National Health Insurance, and other health care measures. The aftermath of the First World War saw a further expansion of this sort of government involvement. The influence of the fourth stage, the Second World War, was not limited to recruits or part of the population, but affected almost every citizen; consequently, health care policy had to broaden to embrace the whole population. And so '... it was necessary for the State to take positive steps in all spheres of the national economy to safeguard the physical health of the people', but this was only part of it, for

> ... it was also an imperative for war strategy for the authorities to concern themselves with that elusive concept 'civilian morale' ... the war could not be won unless millions of ordinary people in Britain and overseas were convinced that we had something better to offer than had our enemies — not only during but after the war. (Titmuss, 1976, p.82)

This chapter is about what happened to health care during the Second World War, and what has happened since. In Britain, a series of events led to the creation of the National Health Service in 1948. The idea of a national health service had been mooted many times previously, and the inter-war period had witnessed a host of detailed proposals, such as the Dawson Report of 1920, successive manifestos of Labour and Liberal parties, and recommendations from the British Medical Association. On the other hand, it must be remembered that the Dawson Report had been shelved within weeks of publication and that other proposals had been largely ignored at the time, coming into their own only during and after the war.

It was in Britain in 1941 that the then Archbishop of Canterbury, Dr Temple, made the first recorded use of the expression the 'welfare state', and in Britain the NHS was one of the forms to be taken by this welfare state. Although things did look very different after the war, how important the war was in the creation of the NHS is a matter of fine judgement and opinion.

In other countries the welfare state took different forms, but the underlying theme was similar: that health care should be seen as a right, like justice and the vote, and that this right could be extended across the population by government involvement in financing and regulating health care. 'Expansion', 'extension', 'growth', 'increase' were the key words in health care occupations, services, and spending. This is not the whole story, however: 'it has been said that armies are always ready to fight the last war, never the next, and the same could be said of the architects of social security systems' (Watkin, 1975, p.73). The post-war health and welfare systems of western Europe and North America were erected on foundations of full employment and economic growth. During the post-war 'long boom', which lasted until the early 1970s, it was not just health care that was growing on an unprecedented scale, so too was the world economy. This is no longer the case; the result is the reopening of a whole series of questions about health and welfare: what is meant by a *right* to health care? How well equipped is the welfare system to deal with changed conditions? How should it adapt?

These are some of the questions to be asked as we consider recent history and the present. How much has really changed, and how new are the problems and dilemmas of the present? Having looked at the past, we are now in a position to begin to draw some lessons from it.

Creating a National Health Service

The National Health Service was devised and created in a period when planning was a dominating feature of Britain's social and economic life. The debates of the 1920s and 1930s about the merits or disadvantages of planning and intervention to tackle unemployment and economic slump were suspended by the Second World War, which forced Britain '... in the interests of survival, into the most state-planned and state-managed economy ever introduced outside a frankly socialist country' (Hobsbawm, 1968, p.208). Such planning was not confined to munitions and armaments production, but penetrated deeply into agriculture and food, housing, the labour market, and, not least, health services.

The most immediate reason for government concern about health services was the fear that bombing would result in mass civilian casualties. Basing calculations on the experiences of bomb casualties during the Spanish Civil War (the 'Barcelona ratio') it had been estimated in 1937 (wrongly, in retrospect) that bombing of Britain would result in 600 000 deaths and twice as many casualties in the first two months of war. In 1938 a committee of eminent psychiatrists had reached the conclusion that 'the conditions of war would so lower the threshold to stress that three to four million acute psychiatric cases could be expected within six months of the outbreak of war' (cited in Jones, 1972, p.271). It seemed essential, therefore, to marshal existing health services into an organisation capable of responding to these threats.

But what were the existing health services? First, there were the hospitals. A survey of the nation's hospitals had fortunately been conducted in 1938 — fortunate because the most recent previous survey had been in 1863! The 1938 survey had revealed around 3 000 hospitals in England as a whole, containing almost 500 000 beds. These hospitals were extraordinarily diverse, but fell into two broad categories: the voluntary hospitals, and the municipal or local authority hospitals. The voluntary hospitals numbered around 1 100 containing 90 000 beds. They included the main teaching hospitals in London and elsewhere, although the typical voluntary hospitals were not large teaching institutions, but rather quite small 'cottage' hospitals, often poorly equipped, badly staffed, and offering care that was often far below the best.

The work of the voluntary hospitals was largely confined to short-term surgical and medical care. Local authority hospitals, particularly in London, provided some acute services, but they also catered for the mentally ill or handicapped, for tuberculosis patients, and for those with infectious diseases. Almost 400 000 beds were in these hospitals; of these almost half were in asylums with the remaining 200 000 largely located in TB sanatoria and isolation hospitals, and in a miscellaneous collection of institutions which were essentially workhouse infirmaries erected under the Poor Law.

Surveying this national stock of hospitals in 1938, therefore, the essential point was that 'there was no hospital system ... there was instead a collection of individual hospitals, criss-crossed, separated, and enclosed by local government boundary barriers, legal, residential and occupational barriers, medical category and financial barriers' (Titmuss, 1976, p.143). In short, the whole collection of hospitals was completely inadequate to the demands of war, and in June 1938 the first step towards a National Health Service was made by creating an Emergency Medical Service.

The Emergency Medical Service reached deep into the running of hospitals: it became closely involved in the finance of over 1 000 of the largest hospitals, containing 300 000 beds; it imposed a regional organisation of twelve

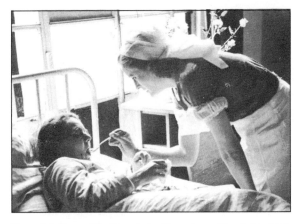

Figure 5.1 'I am a War Nurse'; the Westminster Hospital in 1941, portrayed in *Picture Post*, vol. 13, no. 8, 22 November 1941. The war stimulated a series of long-term changes for nurses: a national negotiating system, recommended rates of pay, recognition of Enrolled or Assistant nurses, and generally improved status. In the words of a *Times* leader in 1941, 'The time has come when all Government Departments must adopt the same attitude to the nursing profession — that it is a profession … Every nurse ought to enjoy a status comparable to that of a commissioned officer; a lower status is detrimental to her service and therefore a handicap upon her patients' (cited in Abel-Smith, 1960, p.165).

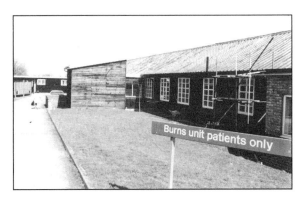

Figure 5.2 Erected under the war-time Emergency Medical Service, these prefabricated buildings are still used by Stoke Mandeville Hospital, Aylesbury.

regions, grouping hospitals by function into casualty clearing hospitals in towns and cities, and treatment and rehabilitation hospitals in the country; it virtually created a general laboratory service, and did create a blood transfusion and ambulance service; it set wages and conditions in the hospitals, erected 1 000 new operating theatres and many thousands of beds in prefabricated annexes, and directed medical staff to areas most in need. And its influence grew as the war progressed: free treatment, '… at first reserved for civilians and military war casualties, was gradually extended to more and more

Table 5.1 Sources of income of London voluntary hospitals, 1938 and 1947 (percentages)

Source of income	Percentage of income in 1938	Percentage of income in 1947
Voluntary gifts	34	16
Investments	16	8
Public Authority payments	8	46
Other payments (patient fees, etc.)	42	30
Total	100	100

(Source: Eckstein, 1958, p.75)

classes of patients — war workers, evacuees, people with fractures, firemen and so on — until a sixty-two page booklet was needed to define the different eligible classes' (Calder, 1971, p.622).

The Emergency Medical Service, for many reasons, was a powerful influence on the shape the NHS took in 1948. First, it gave civil servants and politicians the experience of running a national service. Second, it cruelly exposed the limitations of the previous services. Specialists dispatched as employees of the state from the centres of excellence to the more neglected of the local authority hospitals were confronted with the prevailing standards of hospital care, often for the first time, discovering '… in their general wards an unholy and unhygienic collection of nursing mothers, infants with gastro-enteritis, healthy new-born babies, and aged and chronically sick women' (Titmuss, 1950, p.71). The weak financial basis of the voluntary hospitals was similarly exposed. Table 5.1 shows the changes that occurred in the sources of income of the London voluntary hospitals during the war.

☐ What strikes you as the main change to have occurred during this period?

■ The proportion of the voluntary hospitals' income derived from independent sources collapsed, and the support from public authorities increased sharply.

But perhaps most crucial of all, the Emergency Medical Service provided a large portion of the population for the first time with prompt, free, accessible and good standard medical care — if this were possible in wartime, why not when the peace came also?

Throughout the war years, therefore, the eventual structure of the National Health Service was slowly emerging. One landmark was the publication of the Beveridge Report, containing proposals for a comprehensive social security system that was aimed at overcoming the 'five giants on the road of reconstruction': want, disease, ignorance, squalor and idleness. The attack on disease would be led, assumed the report, by a National

Health Service. Published in December 1942, the report created an enormous surge of popular interest and acclaim:

> outside the shops of His Majesty's Stationery Office, the most significant queues of the war lined up to buy the report. A brief official summary was issued, and sales of the two combined eventually ran to 635 000 copies. Within two weeks of its publication, a Gallup Poll discovered that nineteen people out of twenty had heard of the report, and nine out of ten believed that its proposals should be adopted. (Calder, 1971, p.609)

The period from the publication of the Beveridge Report until the 'Appointed Day' in 1948 when the NHS began work was one of almost continual discussion and argument about the shape the new health service should take, and no group was more deeply involved in this than the doctors.

However, doctors were not a unified group. There were the hospital doctors, whose conditions, career prospects and professional influence all stood to be improved by a National Health Service, as they had already under the Emergency Medical Service. The general practitioners, working largely outside the hospitals, did not all share the same worries: as with the voluntary hospitals, financial problems afflicted large numbers of GPs; young general practitioners were often faced with the problem of having to buy their way into work by purchasing an existing practice for £2 000–3 000, then having to pay off the loan required to do this on an income of perhaps £700 a year. In addition, many GPs, particularly in working-class urban areas, had terms of work that were narrowly tied to conditions laid down by 'approved societies' such as friendly societies and trade unions for whom they provided 'contract practice'. Other GPs, catering for a middle-class clientele, tended to be much better off, and were heavily concentrated in wealthy areas and towns, less loaded with work and therefore more able to devote time to medical politics in the British Medical Association (BMA) and elsewhere. Those who were doing rather better provided the spokespersons for the profession as a whole. We will come to the implications of this shortly.

Apart from finance and divisions of interest, general practice was in poor shape because single-handed practices were the norm: only 10–20 per cent of all GPs were working in group practice. The resulting isolation had resulted in low clinical standards:

> ... the office of an able urban practitioner consisted of two rooms, one for waiting and the other for consultation. There was little to indicate which was which beyond the ancient tilting haircloth examining chair, the wash-basin ... and a few simple instruments which, used for all sorts of purposes,

were never boiled, two or three vials containing mercury or carbolic acid for local applications, and the mantelpiece strewn with proprietary preparations in dust-covered bottles. Urinalysis was employed — but practically no other laboratory procedure. The doctor made up his mind on the basis of symptoms and obvious physical indications. Long experience and natural shrewdness sharpened by necessity carried the best of the old family physicians far ... inability to penetrate beneath the surface constantly forced the practitioner to guess or fumble.

This description, which was cited as 'almost a perfect word-picture' of post-war standards of British general practice according to the highly critical Collings Report of 1950 (Collings, 1950), was in fact a summary of American general practice in the 1880s contained in the Flexner Report on American medical education published in 1911. These then were the formative conditions from which British doctors approached the discussions over a new health service.

The Beveridge Report had lain down the essential principles and objectives of a National Health Service, but it was not until the wartime government published more detailed proposals in a White Paper in 1944 that the political temperature really began to rise. The overall objectives of the new service were simply and clearly expressed:

> To ensure that everybody in the country — irrespective of means, age, sex and occupation — shall have equal opportunity to benefit from the best and most up-to-date medical and allied services available. To provide, therefore, for all who want it, a comprehensive service covering every branch of medical and allied activity.
>
> To divorce the case of health from questions of personal means or other factors irrelevant to it; to provide the service free of charge (apart from certain possible charges in respect of appliances) and to encourage a new attitude to health — the easier obtaining of advice early, the promotion of good health rather than only the treatment of bad. (HMSO, 1944, p.47)

The detailed proposals were for a free and fully comprehensive (or '100 per cent') service, paid for out of central government taxes and local government rates. Hospital doctors would be paid directly for all hospital work they did, and all hospitals — voluntary and local authority — would be administered by 'joint authorities', that is, groups of local authorities joined together to form larger regions. General practitioners would have the choice of continuing in independent practice and being paid by the

Table 5.2 Doctors' responses to the 1944 White Paper (per cent)

Questions	All Pro	All Con	Doctors in Armed Services Pro	Doctors in Armed Services Con	Hospital consultants Pro	Hospital consultants Con	GPs Pro	GPs Con	Salaried doctors in administrative and other posts Pro	Salaried doctors in administrative and other posts Con
For or against White Paper	39	53	53	41	36	58	31	62	60	33
A '100 per cent' service	60	37	73	26	54	44	54	43	74	23
Local authority hospital administration	13	78	13	81	9	84	11	79	24	69
Control over GPs' location	57	39	68	28	56	38	51	45	71	25
Health centres	68	24	83	13	67	23	60	32	84	11
Salaried service in health centres for GPs	62	29	74	20	73	25	53	38	79	22

(Source: derived from Eckstein, 1958, p.148)

capitation system familiar to them under the 1911 Act, or of working in health centres provided by local authorities and receiving a salary. Table 5.2 shows some of the results of a survey conducted in 1944 that asked all doctors what they thought of these proposals.

☐ To what two proposals did all doctors voice the strongest support and objections?
■ There was strong support from all quarters for a health centre policy, but almost outright rejection of the idea that local authorities should be responsible for the hospitals.
☐ On what issues were there significant differences of opinion between the hospital consultants and the GPs?
■ Their reponses were very similar on all major items, although a small majority of GPs was in favour of salaried work in health centres.
☐ How would you describe the general positions of salaried doctors in administration, and doctors in the services, to the proposals?
■ Both groups expressed particularly strong reactions to the proposals, and had majorities in favour of the White Paper as a whole.

The poll had been conducted on behalf of the British Medical Association; but the results were not in line with its policy: the official line was strongly against any form of salaried service, especially if paid through local government. Indeed, far from accepting the results, 'it was now claimed [by the BMA] that the rank and file had not understood the "hidden implications" of the scheme, that the Socialist Medical Association had stuffed the ballot boxes, that salaried doctors should have been excluded from the poll because they had no understanding of private practice' (Eckstein, 1958, p.153). There were still rumblings within the leadership in favour of a '90 per cent' service, in

which the wealthiest 10 per cent of the population would be ineligible for the NHS.

☐ What advantage might a 90 per cent scheme have held for at least some GPs?
■ It would have allowed GPs in wealthier parts of the country to make much better livings than professional colleagues elsewhere by topping up earnings from private practice.

The leadership of the BMA simply were failing to reflect accurately the views of their members as a whole.

In 1945, as the Churchill government was replaced by Attlee's Labour government in a landslide election victory, with Aneurin Bevan appointed as the new Minister of Health, the BMA's intensified campaigning created increasingly deep divisions within the medical profession. The Royal Colleges, representing the views of the hospital doctors, were broadly in support of the proposed NHS, and once their main objection — to the local authority control of hospitals — had been accommodated by a change in Labour policy, their backing went to Bevan rather than the BMA. Bevan's personal qualities undoubtedly were an important factor in carrying the proposals.

None the less, the BMA's campaign against the NHS, and increasingly against Bevan himself, continued until 1948. The final threats of a boycott and even of a campaign of civil disobedience were only quelled when the membership voted with its feet: three months after the 'Appointed Day' on 5 July 1948, 86 per cent of GPs had agreed to work in association with the NHS, the proportion eventually rising to 98 per cent.

The fact that the doctors as a whole only numbered 50 000, or 10 per cent of the half-million people who started working for the NHS in 1948, is easily forgotten when examining the history of this period. But their influence on

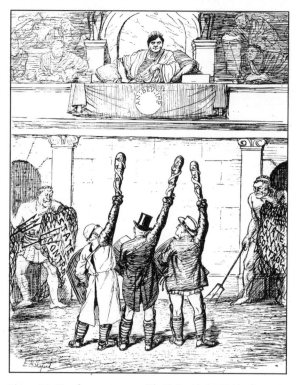

Figure 5.3 *Punch* not unexpectedly sided with the BMA, shown in this cartoon being forced by the gladiators of state control to pay homage to 'Emperor' Bevan.

the structure and workings of the NHS was out of all proportion to their numbers. This can be seen in the main features of the NHS in 1948. The NHS was administered after 1948 by three sets of bodies subject to varying degrees of control and direction from the Ministry of Health: one set dealt with hospitals, another with non-hospital, dental and ophthalmic services and the third with the services provided by local authorities. This three-way administrative division of services is normally referred to as the 'tripartite structure' of the NHS at that time.

Hospitals

Following the Act of 1946 virtually all hospitals in Britain were nationalised; the total number in England was around 3 000, and only some 200, mainly very small nursing homes or religious hospitals, were exempted. The reasons for nationalisation were partly based on ethical arguments:

> ... as the parliamentary debates indicate, many Labour MPs found the voluntary hospital system morally obnoxious, particularly due to the repellent practices used in the latter days of the system to extract money from the public: stunt appeals, bridge tournaments, flag days, midnight matinees, and soap

sales, and not least, the sale of advertising space on hospital walls to patent medicine manufacturers. (Eckstein, 1958, p.178)

But managerial arguments were uppermost: a nationalised system of hospitals, it was argued, would allow more rational planning and control. The first step was to create fourteen (later fifteen) Regional Hospital Boards (RHBs) to plan and supervise hospital services in each region. One 'irrational' element in this was that the teaching hospitals were not placed under RHB control, but were allowed independent Boards of Governors: twenty-six of the thirty-six Boards of Governors were in London, and thus the old divisions between the élite voluntary hospitals and other hospitals were not immediately dissolved.

Detailed administration within each RHB was placed in the hands of almost 400 Hospital Management Committees (HMCs) organised such that each HMC ran a group of hospitals providing a full range of hospital services. Some 'groups' were a single, large, general hospital, others contained more than fifteen small, specialist or physically scattered hospitals that, taken together, would be seen as in some sense equivalent to a single, large, general hospital. Grouping, therefore, was not seen as ideal, but rather as 'a makeshift arrangement pending the construction of an adequate system of general hospitals, forced upon the service by the state of the old hospital system' (Eckstein, 1958, p.158).

Membership of the Regional Hospital Boards was by the appointment of the Minister of Health; RHB members in turn appointed people to the Hospital Management Committees. Table 5.3 shows some characteristics of these memberships in 1952.

☐ How would you summarise the pattern shown in Table 5.3?

Table 5.3 Membership of RHBs and HMCs in 1952

Sex	RHBs	HMCs
Men	85	77
Women	15	23
Occupation		
Doctor/dentist	29	27
Other professions	23	9
Industry and commerce	13	17
Manual workers	3	6
Others (independent, retired, etc.)	32	41
Previous hospital experience		
Yes	85	76
No	15	24

(Source: derived from Eckstein, 1958, p.188)

■ Membership of both RHBs and HMCs was (i) predominantly male; (ii) predominantly professional with very few manual workers; and (iii) mainly composed of people with past experience of hospital administration.

Membership was on a voluntary, unpaid basis, and this in part explains the predominance of people with means and time to take office.

Executive Councils

To administer the services of general medical and dental practitioners, and certain ophthalmic and pharmaceutical services, 138 Executive Councils were created, each covering the approximate area of local authorities. Again, rational management was a central objective of the arrangements, but in practice the new arrangement for providers of these services was similar to the pre-war arrangements: medical practitioners received capitation payments in much the same way as they had since 1911; dentists, chemists, ophthalmologists and opticians could continue to practise wherever they wished, and simply received a fee for each item of service provided to an NHS patient. An important part of the Executive Councils' work, therefore, was simply to administer the pay and work of practitioners and keep records, rather than to plan, in any interventionist sense, these non-hospital health services.

Local authority services

One reason why the Executive Councils did not have this planning function was that they did not have the power or the money to build the series of health centres that would have allowed doctors, dentists, opticians and others to be brought together in planned locations. The health centres were to have been provided by the local authorities, along with environmental health services, maternity and child welfare services, home helps, ambulance services, health visitors and other aspects of domiciliary care. However, because the money for a comprehensive health centre construction programme was not forthcoming, the task of integrating the tripartite system of the NHS was made considerably more difficult. Integration became a constant theme of proposals to reorganise the system.*

The creation of the NHS marked a huge political change, and the financial basis and control of health care were transformed. But in administrative terms, as we have seen, there was much continuity with the past. In the fabric of the health service the continuity of the NHS was even more striking. Table 5.4 shows some results of a survey, conducted in 1953, of the hospital stock of the NHS.

□ What strikes you in this table?
■ The proportion of all the hospitals inherited by the NHS that dated from the nineteenth century was high — almost one half. But the proportion of mental hospitals that were old or very old was substantially higher.

'The Victorians could not build other than solidly, and there the buildings stand, grim, almost indestructible, and they constitute the majority of our mental hospital accommodation', said Kenneth Robinson MP in 1954 during the first parliamentary debate on mental health for twenty-four years. And a few years later, at the 1961 Annual Conference of the National Association for Mental Health (MIND), the Minister for Health, Enoch Powell, returned to the same theme: 'There they stand, isolated, majestic, imperious, brooded over by the gigantic water-tower and chimney combined, rising unmistakeable and daunting out of the countryside — the asylums which our forefathers built with such immense solidity. Do not for a moment underestimate their power of resistance to our assault' (cited in Jones, 1972, p.322).

Nor was the age of the hospital stock the only legacy of the past. In 1948, glaring disparities existed in different parts of the UK as to the health services available. Doctors and dentists were concentrated in areas where the opportunities for private practice were greatest, in voluntary hospitals where endowments and bequests had been most forthcoming, and in municipal hospitals where

*A brief account of changes in the NHS's structure, and a much fuller analysis of its current structure and operation, are contained in The Open University (1985) *Caring for Health: Dilemmas and Prospects*, The Open University Press (U205 *Health and Disease*, Book VIII).

Table 5.4 The age of hospitals in England and Wales (in 1953)

Hospital buildings originally erected before:	Total (%)	Mental Illness and Mental Deficiency (%)	Other (%)
1891	45	65	43
1861	21	40	18

(Source: Abel-Smith and Titmuss, 1954, p.54, Table 34)

local authorities had high rate incomes or particular enthusiasm for hospital building.

Finally, it was not entirely clear who was going to reap most benefit from the NHS. As a measure designed to provide free and universal access to health care, the assumption was, and largely still is, that the NHS would bring particular benefits to the working class.

☐　But think back to the descriptions of hospitals in the previous chapter. Who mainly used them, and who mainly didn't use them until the twentieth century?
■　On the whole, hospitals were lower-class institutions until the twentieth century. The middle classes made much less use of them.

In 1958 the American political scientist Harry Eckstein, in one of the best studies of the formation of the NHS, argued that 'the social distribution of the British medical services before the Appointed Day was biased very much in favour of the lower classes' (apart from the general practitioner services and dental and optical services); and that '... the medico-economic problems of the poor were attributable to their general conditions of life rather than to the inaccessibility of medical services. From a purely economic standpoint, then, the National Health Service was bound to be a middle-class more than a lower-class service. Indeed, some of the innovations made by the service (for example, improvements in the physical layout and organization of hospital out-patient departments) are comprehensible only in these terms' (Eckstein, 1958, pp.9 and 43). Universal access, on this account, meant increased access for the middle classes.

So the age, design, location and class distribution of the health care services and institutions brought into the NHS all continued to exert powerful influences. The NHS might have been a new start but it had inherited a legacy that was to dictate many of its policies, circumscribe many of its actions, and pose many of its problems in future years.*

Years of growth

The formation of the NHS was a unique historical event, but in many other respects the post-war development of health care in Britain was influenced by forces also affecting all other industrial countries. As we reach the end of this historical account and begin to turn to a wider international perspective, let us begin by noting some common themes in Britain and elsewhere.

Not only in Britain but elsewhere, government increased its involvement in the provision of health care.

*A detailed account of the post-1948 development of the NHS is provided in *Caring for Health: Prospects and Dilemmas* (U205 *Health and Disease*, Book VIII).

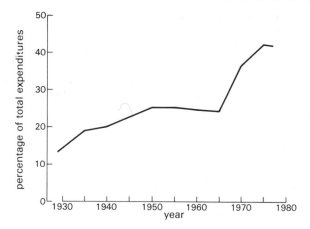

Figure 5.4 The public-sector share of the total health care budget, USA, 1929–1977 (%)
(Source: Maxwell, 1981, Figure 4.2, p.62)

This involvement took many different forms, some of which are examined in more detail in Chapter 8, but the basic theme was one of growth. Figure 5.4 shows the way in which the government share of total health care expenditure in the United States changed between 1929 and 1977.

This growing involvement of government in the provision of health care has gone further in most west European countries, as Table 5.5 shows.

☐　What reasons can you think of for the increasing involvement of government in providing health care? (You might think back to the discussion of the Poor Law medical services in Chapter 4.)

Table 5.5 Public expenditure as a percentage of total expenditure on health in ten European countries 1962–1974

Country	Public expenditure (percentages) in:	
	1962	1974
Austria	63	65
Belgium	72	84
Finland	64	95
France	66	77
West Germany	55	78
Greece	64	66
Netherlands	64	70
Norway	73	95
Sweden	77	92
Switzerland	53	70

(Source: WHO, 1981)

■ One fundamental reason was to extend access to health care services by filling the gaps left by the market, by charity or by self-help.

Growing provision of health care by governments in post-war years was only part of a general trend towards state intervention in many other areas of economy and society. And the post-war period also witnessed a surge in state interest in environmental and public health. The nineteenth-century sanitary and environmental reform movement had undoubtedly led to improvement in the European countries and the USA, but the Second World War itself had caused immense damage, existing regulations were often poorly enforced and new health hazards were to become apparent.

Housing was an immediate concern of many European countries and the programmes that ensued brought modern sewage systems and water supplies where none had existed previously, saw the first effective reduction in overcrowding and involved the state on a larger scale than hitherto in the provision of housing. In Britain, for example, in the ten years immediately after the war two million new homes were built, five-eighths of them by local authorities, and overcrowding began to decrease. The number of persons per room in Britain, for instance, fell from 0.83 in 1931 to 0.66 in 1961.

One of the most tangible manifestations of continued environmental health hazards was the recurrence of appalling winter smogs. In Pennsylvania in 1948, the Donora fog prompted a major public enquiry and led to some tightening of existing regulations. Then in December 1952 a dense fog in London was associated with an excess mortality of 4 000 deaths in the smog area in the first three weeks in December.

There were many factors contributing to the lack of effective action on atmospheric pollution. In the nineteenth century smoke was considered to be a glorious sign of industrial progress. As one member of the Darlington Board of Health argued in 1866:

If I go to Middlesbrough I see large works ... sending out thousands and thousands of cubic feet of gas and smoke ... I ask the individuals who live there if they do not suffer in their health. They say, 'No, it is all good for trade, we want more of it, we find no fault with smoke'. (Cited in Wohl, 1983, p.216)

Until the twentieth century the possible threat in many countries to industry and employment meant that regulations were constantly evaded, the standard legislative escape clause being that they should only be taken 'as far as is practicable having regard to the nature of the manufacture or trade'. Fines remained ineffectively low, being set at a mere £50 maximum in England, for example, after the 1936 Public Health Act. Nearly half of all smoke

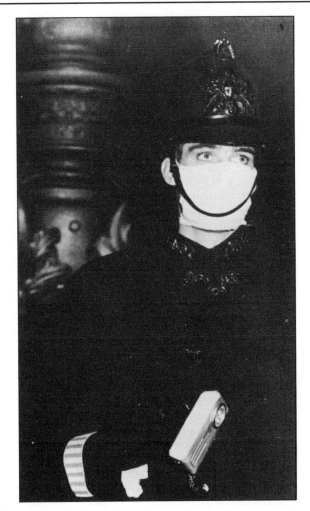

Figure 5.5 A London smog in the 1950s. Police on duty were forced to wear smog masks.

pollution arose from domestic chimneys, yet in most countries at the end of the 1940s there was no control in this area. In Britain it was the 'killer fog' in London from 5–9 December 1952 which eventually brought smoke abatement to the forefront of the public mind, where it remained by constant pressure from the National Society for Smoke Abatement and from a large group of MPs and a few committed Medical Officers of Health, until the Clean Air Act of 1956 was passed. This Act established smokeless zones and for the first time domestic smoke emissions were brought under control.

The difficulties of extending comprehensive environmental and public health controls to industry were caused partly by fundamental changes taking place in the structure of European and American industry. Processes which in the pre-war period had been used only on a laboratory scale became major new industrial practices; those in the nuclear and petrochemical industries are two of the most striking examples. The speed of these changes often outstripped the institutions, regulations and technologies required to control and monitor them, as a catalogue of major industrial incidents testifies. In Japan, these included the Minamata episode, when forty-five people died from organic mercury poisoning after eating contaminated fish, the Itai-Itaibyo Episode ('*itai-itai*' means 'extreme pain') when fifty-six deaths occurred from cadmium poisoning in water and farm products, and Yokkaichi Episode, when 451 people contracted chronic asthma from sulphur emissions from an oil refinery. Each country has its own list: in Britain Aberfan in 1966 and Flixborough in 1974, and so on. Some have been international in their consequences, like the thalidomide tragedy in 1963.

The legislation that has ensued to strengthen control incorporates a number of common principles. Government agencies consolidating existing provision and enforcing common standards have been set up — the Health and Safety Executive in Britain and The Environmental Protection Agency in the USA. Responsibility for preventing industrial hazards and sickness has been seen increasingly to lie with employers, who have also been required to inform both workers and the surrounding community of the potential hazards of the production processes involved. Powers of enforcement have been increased, licensing systems extended and legislation in the form of 'enabling Acts' more widely used. The last is essentially an Act which sets a framework within which codes of practice, regulations and 'safe' standards can be regularly amended as technology and research develop.

Public and environmental health has had to try to adapt to constant and rapid technological change. In personal health care, too, a whole host of changes have resulted from technical innovations. First, new technology has given rise to new occupations in health care. For example, heart-lung machines, which have made many heart operations possible, require 'pump technicians'. The widespread use of audiometers to test children's hearing has given rise to specialised audiometricians. And perhaps the largest growth area in hospital staff has been the vast increase in the number of medical laboratory scientific officers. For example, every general hospital now has a laboratory to investigate viral infections, using technology that has been developed over the past forty years.

The second change has been in the content of some health workers' jobs. In many maternity hospitals, midwives have had to become familiar with electronic equipment and machinery to pump synthetic hormones into women in labour — a sharp contrast to clean towels and lots of hot water! Such changes have led to concern that doctors, nurses, midwives and others have started to pay more attention to the machines than to the patient.

The introduction of so much new technology into hospitals has led to the third change, that of the architecture and atmosphere of the buildings. Increasing amounts of space are taken up with machinery and associated activities, with the consequence that the space occupied by patients and beds in a modern hospital is often less than in a nineteenth-century building. This has happened for a number of reasons. One is the increasing amount of administration in contemporary health care: as doctors have become more specialised in their work, it has become necessary for an increasing number of different specialists to be involved in the care of an individual patient. Before 1940 a general physician would have looked after all aspects of the care and management of a patient. Now, because of specialisation, it has become essential to ensure an accurate and reliable means of communication between the various doctors that may be involved, and the main vehicle for this is the patient's medical record, which has grown from just a few pages to a file which in some instances is several inches thick. So records departments, and the people to maintain them, have come to take up an increasing amount of hospital space.

One objective of some post-war technology has been to speed up tasks, such as the chemical analysis of blood and urine. Not only has this affected the content of the work which laboratory technicians do; it has also affected the volume of work. It has permitted the establishment of various screening procedures; for instance, the testing of vast numbers of people who are not complaining of any specific medical problems, such as the testing of all new-born babies for phenylketonuria — a condition which if ignored will result in mental retardation — which has been made possible by automated laboratory testing equipment.

All the trends discussed so far have tended to be increases rather than decreases in health care activities and facilities. In contrast, one of the most dramatic changes resulting from technology has been a reduction in the number of people confined to psychiatric hospitals as a result of new drugs, in particular a group known as the major tranquillisers. While there is considerable debate about the extent to which such drugs are 'medical straight-jackets', their introduction and use has certainly led to a massive reduction in the number of psychiatric in-patients. Similarly, other new drugs have led to changes in the use of hospitals. Some of the new anaesthetic agents mean that patients feel well enough to go home within hours rather than days of an operation. Similarly, antibiotics have reduced the problem of infections after operations, and thus contributed to a reduction in the length of time people need to stay in hospital.

All change?

Although only a few examples of the impact of technology have been mentioned, it should be clear that it is a potent factor affecting the pattern of health care, and is likely to become more so in the future. Technological change takes its place alongside industrial change, demographic change, scientific change, social change, religious change, and epidemiological change, all of which have figured large in the book so far. Change seems to be one of the few constants in the history of health care, although some would dispute even this on the grounds that the pace of change is greater than ever before:

> ... the only event historically comparable to the Industrial Revolution is the Neolithic Revolution. But apart from every other consideration, the Neolithic Revolution developed in the course of thousands of years. It took more than 5000 years to move from the Middle East to Scandinavia ... The Industrial Revolution has invaded the world, turned our very existence upside down and overthrown the structures of all existing human societies in the course of only eight generations. And today it is beginning to press with great urgency new problems of such enormity that the human mind can hardly grasp them — the uncontrolled increase in population; the hydrogen bomb; the pollution of the atmosphere, the destruction of the natural surroundings by industrial waste; the demand for further mass education; the presence of an ever-increasing number of old people kept alive but rejected by the rest of society; the breaking up of the traditional state; the scientific organisation of uncontrolled centres of power; the unlimited possibilities held out by geneticists and biologists of influencing nature and ... behaviour ... Under the weight of these problems the old structures crumble ... Everyone has been taken by surprise. (Cipolla, 1976a, pp.20–1)

However, as the creation of the NHS illustrated, the past is often present in many powerful ways, exerting influences through ideas and institutions, buildings and customs, practices and people. It is possible on this account to make a decisive break with the past in some respects, but not to abolish or ignore it.

Objectives for Chapter 5

When you have studied this chapter, you should be able to:

5.1 Discuss the ways in which health care has been influenced by wars, with particular reference to Britain during the Second World War.

5.2 Outline the position of the medical profession towards proposals for a National Health Service.

5.3 Describe some key aspects of change and continuity represented by the NHS.

5.4 Identify international similarities in post-war health care.

Questions for Chapter 5

1 (*Objective 5.1*) '... not until three years had passed, and victory was at last a rational — rather than an emotional — concept, could the enemy claim that he had killed as many British soldiers as women and children' (Titmuss, 1976, p.82). What might you infer from this comment on the Second World War about likely developments in health and social policy?

2 (*Objective 5.2*) What were the main divisions of opinion among doctors towards the NHS?

3 (*Objective 5.3*) 'The National Health Service Act made no new resources available for health care, for many years it built no new hospitals, and the training of doctors and nurses went on much as before, without any positive intervention by the Government' (Watkin, 1975, pp.137–8). Give some examples of the types of pre-war patterns of health care resources inherited by the NHS.

4 (*Objective 5.4*) How would you characterise the development of public and environmental health measures in post-war industrial countries?

6

Lay
health care in
contemporary
Britain

During this chapter you will be referred to the Course Reader for the article 'Caring for the Spouse who Died', written by Ann Bowling and Ann Cartwright (Part 6, Section 6.5).

The fundamental importance of the lay health care sector was clearly stated in Chapter 1. And yet, because of its major absence from both the historical record and from historical research, relatively little attention has so far been paid to it. Now that the story has reached present times, however, it is at last possible to say something more systematic.

Although research vividly demonstrates the continuing importance of lay care, there are still large gaps in what is known. Most research into health care still focuses on formal and professional care, and that which does examine the lay sector has some major omissions — we know, for example, very little about people's own views of the lay care they receive from others, or about lay care in the Third World. None the less, there is still much that can be said, though our focus here will be almost entirely on Britain, a country where lay health care has been the subject of rather more research than many others.

This chapter addresses two key aspects of contemporary British lay health care in some detail. The first section of the chapter is descriptive. It concerns questions such as these: just how big is the lay sector? What is the demand for such care? What kinds of care are undertaken in the lay sector? Just who is it that provides this care? And what are the financial costs of actually doing such work?

The second part of the chapter turns from description to debate. The relationship between lay and formal care has always been controversial. What is the nature of the boundary between the two? How far should the state or the medical professions intervene, aid and supervise lay care? Or how far, instead, should people look after their own health, using doctors only in an ancillary capacity? As you will see, all these questions are still central to the modern debate.

Contemporary lay care: an overview

☐ Chapters 2–4 have described several developments that may have transferred activities between informal and formal care. What examples can you think of?

■ Some of the major developments were: first, the creation and huge elaboration of special institutions — hospitals, poorhouses, or asylums — whose populations included sick people previously cared for at home; second, the creation and, over the last century, massive expansion of medical services for the poor who might not otherwise have been able to afford the services of a practitioner; third, the development of pensions, accident benefits, insurance, and other forms of social security providing sources of aid besides the family.

For all the extraordinary elaboration of formal health care services and despite the fact that the number of kinship ties have undoubtedly lessened (although some would argue that the *quality* may have increased), it remains the case, as you will now see, that the lay health care sector is still of fundamental importance; so much so, indeed, that it should undoubtedly be called the 'primary health care sector' — were it not for the fact that general practitioners and health visitors have already grabbed this title for themselves.

To understand the continuing fundamental importance of lay care, begin by considering Table 6.1, which is based on health diaries kept by seventy-nine London women over a six-week period.

☐ What does the table suggest about the relation of formal medical services to the most common symptoms of illness?

■ That most symptoms of illness are not the subject of formal medical consultation — even a sore throat, the

Table 6.1 Symptom episodes and medical consultations recorded in health diaries kept by 79 women aged 16–44 years

Ten most frequent symptoms	Ratio of consultations to symptom episodes
Tiredness, lack of energy	no consultations
Nerves, depression or irritability	1:74
Headache	1:60
Backache	1:38
Sleeplessness	1:31
Muscle and joint aches and pains	1:18
Cold or flu	1:12
Stomach pains	1:11
Women's complaints (e.g. period pain)	1:10
Sore throat	1:9

(Source: derived from Scambler, *et al*, 1981, pp.746–50)

least common of the ten, was the subject of consultation in only one case for every nine cases reported.

☐ What does this also reveal about diagnosis?

■ That diagnosis is as much a matter for the laity as it is for the professionals; indeed, simply to reach professional care, lay diagnostic decisions must usually be made.*

Lay diagnosis is more than a matter of individual decision making. Just as there is now a highly developed professional referral system in which patients are transferred from one specialist to another, so too there is, as there always has been, a *lay referral system*, in which members of the laity consult health care books for themselves or consult with one another, not just with doctors (the term is that of Eliot Freidson, an American sociologist (1960)). More detailed research has begun into this area — though like the rest of lay care, there is still much that has not been investigated.

Not surprisingly, people use a wide variety of sources of information in making up their minds what to do about symptoms. In a study conducted in 1971, Christopher Elliot-Binns, a British general practitioner, found that half of a sample of 1 000 patients using his surgery had decided to treat themselves prior to consulting a paid medical practitioner: 88 per cent had received advice from others before attending and a few had tapped five or more different sources of information. The advice came predominantly from friends 50 per cent), spouses (47 per cent) and other relatives (38 per cent). Magazines and books were consulted by 16 per cent, though the home medical manuals that were used were rather old — 27 years on average (Elliot-Binns, 1973).

Very different advice seemed to come from different sorts of people. Elliot-Binns found that wives were much more likely to offer reassurance and comfort to their husbands, while, faced with their wife's symptoms, husbands were more likely to suggest formal medical consultation. Another study by Annette Scambler, a psychologist, and her colleagues, has suggested that the route to lay or professional care also depends on wider links to family and friends (Scambler, Scambler and Craig, 1981). Women in close contact with their mothers were more likely to consult their general practitioner; those with lots of female friends seemed to redefine their symptoms as less important.

So a central part of lay health care is not just diagnosing illness in oneself but being prepared to offer diagnostic

*The problems and techniques of lay diagnosis and their resemblance to those of professional practitioners are discussed in The Open University (1985) *Experiencing and Explaining Disease*, Chapter 2, The Open University Press (U205 *Health and Disease*, Book VI).

advice, where necessary, to others. That advice, as often as not, is to do nothing or to treat oneself. Again, relatively little research has been done into lay methods of treatment. One obvious recourse, however, is the many traditional remedies that still survive.

☐ Write down some folk remedies of which you are aware.
■ You may have thought of:
hot toddy for colds and flu
copper bracelets for rheumatism
brown sugar and onion juice for bronchitis
vinegar and brown paper ironed on the back for lumbago
dock leaves for stings
milkweed for warts
gold wedding ring rubbed on sties

Whatever the extent of traditional remedies, self-medication using proprietary medicines* is also of major importance. In the UK a major study was undertaken in 1969 by two sociologists, Karen Dunnel and Ann Cartwright. Eighty per cent of a large sample of the population drawn from right across the country said they had taken some medicine in the two weeks prior to the interview. Self-prescribed medicines — such as aspirin, tonics, skin preparations and antacids — outnumbered those prescribed by doctors by two to one.

Another indication of the extent of self-medication is the amount spent each year on 'over-the-counter' proprietary medicines, which are available without need of a doctor's prescription. In 1980–1981 £426 million was spent in the UK on these and on other self-prescribed medical goods.

Not only are most symptoms diagnosed and treated solely by the laity but vast amounts of health maintenance work is a lay not professional task. The Hippocratic and medieval emphasis on diet, rest, exercise and so forth is still with us, but in addition there are other tasks. Consider Figure 6.1.

☐ What does this suggest about health and housework?
■ That a lot of what we conventionally think of as housework — an activity which annually involves billions of woman-hours — also has an important health maintenance aspect. Keeping things clean is not necessarily just a matter of neatness, ritual or respectability; it can also have an important preventive health aspect, and the same is true of the preparation of food.

*Medicines whose manufacture and sale are covered by patent laws.

10 POINT CODES FOR HOUSEWIVES

1 Buy only from clean places. Get the food home clean.

2 Use clean containers in your home. Use your refrigerator properly. If in doubt, find out.

3 Keep family foods away from food for pets. Use separate utensils and crockery.

4 Wash your hands always before preparing food, always after using the W.C. See your children do too.

5 Cover cuts and sores with waterproof dressings. If you are not well with no one to take your place in the kitchen then be extra careful about personal cleanliness.

6 Keep food clean, covered and either cool or piping hot.

7 Reheated leftovers must be made really hot right through. Do the same with ready packed foods intended to be eaten hot.

8 Keep working surfaces clean. Use really hot, soapy water. A wipe with a dish cloth is not enough.

9 Stack washed and rinsed crockery and pans to drain. If you use drying cloths be sure they are clean.

10 Keep the lid on the dustbin.

HEALTH EDUCATION COUNCIL

Figure 6.1 Advice sheet issued by the Health Education Council in 1984.

☐ What is the historical origin of these rules?
■ Some have probably been around in one form or another for a very long time, but many stem primarily from the nineteenth century: from the initial desire to develop sanitary conditions, and from later nineteenth-century microbiology and germ theory. Such ideas were then popularised in many different ways: at a personal level by health visitors, and also through pamphlets, magazines, adverts, religion and entertainment. Our present ideas and rules are equally ubiquitous.

Finally, for all the growth of hospitals, asylums and so forth, as well as the development of a vast formal nursing sector, most nursing is still done primarily by family members. Not only has there been a recent trend away from institutional care, but, as we have already seen, the vast array of everyday symptoms are treated largely at home.

Considerable lay nursing care must be provided for many acute conditions such as colds, flu and childhood measles. The same is true for the management of many chronic conditions such as diabetes — such care may indeed be the major determinant of outcome. In addition,

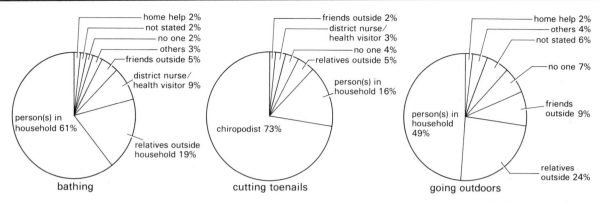

Figure 6.2 Sources of help for various domestic activities of the elderly. (NB The percentage totals are slightly high because the figures have been rounded up)
(Source: based on data in Hunt, 1978, from a sample of 2 622 people aged 65 or over in 1 975 households.)

there have been major demographic shifts which have led to a strikingly new pattern of lay nursing.

□ How might recent demographic changes have affected the pattern of lay nursing?
■ On the one hand, the birth rate is much lower and those children that are born are far healthier — so the amount of child care and child nursing has dramatically lessened. But this has been matched at the other end of the life-cycle by a huge growth in the proportion of elderly people in the population with a corresponding major rise in the need for nursing care.*

□ What change in state policy might, nevertheless, have led to extra work as regards child care?
■ Many European states, particularly from the end of the nineteenth century, prompted by military and industrial competition, became increasingly concerned about the quality as well as the quantity of babies. There was therefore a major state effort to raise what were seen as the low standards of care for the young.

So despite the major quantitative decline of child care for the lay sector, extra demands were also placed on it. None the less, it is probably in the area of care for the elderly that the most rapidly increasing demands have come. While not all elderly people are in need of such care, it has been estimated that 21 per cent of people over 65 in private households are moderately incapacitated and 10 per cent severely so — amounting in all to some 2.5 million people in the UK. Some indication of the extent to which such care is provided by lay sources is given in Figure 6.2 which is based on a survey of the elderly at home conducted by Audrey Hunt (Hunt, 1978).

*These demographic changes are discussed in detail in *The Health of Nations, ibid.* (U205 Book III).

□ Comment briefly on the pattern of care illustrated in Figure 6.2.
■ Lay sources of care — household members, relatives outside the household and friends — are the most important sources of care in all instances except the cutting of toe nails.

Lay nursing is frequently undertaken willingly and lovingly, but it can involve considerable direct and indirect costs for those providing the care. Direct costs may be associated with special diets, laundry requirements, extra heating costs, transport costs or the costs of adapting dwellings. Providing lay health care of this type may also mean partial loss of income and employment because hours of work need to be changed or reduced, or employment given up altogether. There may also sometimes be profound stress:

Because he had a stroke, he couldn't speak at all and I sound like a gibbering maniac when I get with anyone who can hold a conversation. And then it's back home to talking to myself again. (Wife caring for husband)

They progress in spasms ... It's terribly depressing when you get the same gibberish every day, not even a new sound. You don't want words, you just want a new sound and you don't get anything for weeks and you begin to think 'Is all this teaching worth it?' (Mother of two-year-old deaf child) (Both cited in Finch and Groves, 1983, pp.81 and 55)

Much of the writing on lay nursing care therefore paints a rather gloomy picture of the considerable burden that it can impose and of the responsibilities involved. However, it is also clear that many people do not give up their independence easily and that many caring situations are reciprocal, with, for example, elderly people providing childcare and doing simple household tasks, while younger people go out to work.

Let's now briefly review the scope of the entire lay sector. What have we seen? For all the huge growth of hospitals and for all the enormous development of formal health care occupations, an examination of diagnosis, treatment, health maintenance and ordinary nursing care suggests that in all these areas lay care is still of central, often primary, importance. Doctors, nurses, ambulances and hospitals are the publicly visible aspects of health care. Precisely because of that, it is tempting to assume that they must be the most important. The reverse, however, is the real truth. Health care is like an iceberg — only a very small part floats above the surface of public life. The visible part rests on a far larger but normally submerged basis. Moreover, that basis, as we shall now see, is submerged in yet another way.

The division of labour in lay health care

There are two central points to be remembered about lay health care. The first, as we have just seen, is that the lay sector is far larger than that staffed by professionals. The second is that the vast amount of work involved in that sector is far from equally distributed: the overwhelming amount of work in the lay sector is done by women. Health care is one of the main areas in social life where gender differences are at their most rigid. Consider the following range of research findings. A study of just over 1 000 consultations in well-baby and paediatric clinics in Aberdeen found that on only eighteen occasions was the father the child's sole representative in the clinic. Children were almost always accompanied by mothers, not fathers. Even where both parents have paid jobs, the same rule seems to apply. A survey of 400 couples in which both' partners had medical careers found that 80 per cent of the men held that it was their wife's responsibility to look after the children when they were sick. A similar division of labour is found at the other end of the life-cycle. In a recent study of 22 families caring for severely disabled, elderly relatives, researchers Muriel Nissel and Lucy Bonnerjea estimated that on average 3 hours 24 minutes a day were spent in caring work, and of this only 13 minutes involved husbands — all the rest was done by wives (Nissel and Bonnerjea, 1982). In every aspect of lay health care, whether it be diagnosis, treatment, health maintenance or nursing care, it is mainly women who are expected to do the work and, by and large, actually do so. It is women mostly who buy home health manuals, it is women who do the health maintenance of housework and food preparation, and it is towards women that much official health propaganda is directed (see Figure 6.1). Consider the following quotations which have been taken from, in turn,

an American research unit, a commercially sponsored campaign, and a government report:

> Education has an important impact on maternal capabilities — a mother's ability to do her job. It increases her skills, her knowledge and her ability to deal with new ideas ... Better information about nutrition and hygiene can lead directly to prevention of some of the most common childhood diseases ... Education enables a mother to meet the challenges of a hazardous environment more successfully. (*Worldwatch*, 1981, pp.27 and 29)

> It is highly unlikely that you will persuade your husband to give up smoking if you smoke yourself; show your husband that you intend to deal firmly with the smoking habit ... The sensible wife will first decide whether her husband should lose weight and then plan his menu accordingly ... let your husband talk about his worries and wherever possible take the work from him — draft letters, pay bills, arrange for the plumber yourself ... (Flora Margarine Project for Heart Disease Prevention)

> Services should not only be available to parents but they should be easy to use ... It is a question of, for example, organising child health clinics at times which are convenient for mothers ... (HMSO, 1976, para. 5.9, p.86)

□ Comment briefly on whose health women are assumed to be responsible for, and how.

■ According to these extracts, women are assumed to have specific responsibility for the health of children and husbands, and more generally for the health of the family, whoever that includes. This responsibility is to be exercised through a mother's control of standards of nutrition and hygiene, through the good example they should set for others with regard to individual behaviour and through reducing the pressure on other family members, notably the husband — by both taking over 'his' work and by providing emotional support, i.e. someone to talk to. Women are also assumed to be responsible for the use of health services, particularly child health services.

As the quotations below suggest, women themselves usually accept such responsibility, but they also illustrate the limits of women's 'control' over other members of the family:

> I try and give them a good staple diet. If they like just vegetables you're on a winner but you can't force them to eat it ...

> I try and cut down his potatoes ... I don't tell him

but he gets up from the table and eats bread instead. (Farrant and Russell, 1985)

So, responsibility for health maintenance falls largely on women, and so too does the responsibility for nursing care. A national survey conducted for the Department of Employment in 1980 studied the working lives of roughly five and a half thousand women aged between sixteen and fifty-nine (Martin and Roberts, 1984). No less than one in seven of these women were currently caring for someone 'such as a sick or elderly friend or member of the family who depended on them to provide some regular service in addition to looking after the family in the normal way'. Sixty-eight per cent of such women were caring for a parent or parent-in-law and 84 per cent of them were married, so they probably also had a wide range of domestic health responsibilities at home.

Such responsibilities may have serious effects on women's income and employment prospects. Research has tried to estimate how much income is thereby lost. In the twenty-two families in Muriel Nissel's and Lucy Bonner-jea's study, for example, the loss of earnings in 1982 of those who gave up work was £4 500 per annum on average, and for those who worked reduced hours the figure was £1 900. In another survey of families caring for disabled children, conducted in 1981 it was also found that around £2 000 per annum was lost on average because of a reduction or a change in hours of employment. In both studies the vast majority of those giving up or reducing hours of work were the women in the families.

Given the major financial problems that lay nursing care can produce, some countries have introduced cash payments to compensate lay carers for their loss of earnings. However, such public provision frequently excludes married women — unpaid nursing care is simply assumed to be part of the married woman's duties. Thus in the United Kingdom the Invalid Care Allowance which was introduced in 1975 is available at present only to men and to single women who have given up full-time paid work in order to look after a severely disabled person. Married and cohabiting women are excluded because, according to the Department of Health and Social Security, they have 'the support of their partner's income' (DHSS Evidence to the National Insurance Advisory Committee, 1980, para. 16, p.6). In consequence, the Invalid Care Allowance is only paid to a tiny minority of those engaged in such care. By 1981, six years after the beginning of the scheme, only 6 500 people were in receipt of this benefit.

The size of the lay sector of health care and the gender division of labour are both topics forming part of a study published in 1982 by two medical sociologists, Ann Bowling and Ann Cartwright. Their study focused on the experiences and attitudes of about 360 elderly widowed men and women, their general practitioners and their relatives, friends and neighbours. Part of this study is included in the Course Reader* and you should read this article now, before considering the following questions.

☐ What evidence does 'Caring for the Spouse who Died' give about the scale of lay care?

■ In the sample, almost one-half of deaths occurred at home, and almost one-half had needed help at home with dressing, undressing and bathing.

☐ Were the symptoms of ill-health that spouses had to deal with generally minor?

■ No, some were very serious: examples included constant vomiting, choking or incontinence, and quite violent 'brain storms'.

☐ How would you summarise the effects of providing lay care on the social activities and finances of the carers?

■ 53 per cent of carers had had to give up some activities, a proportion that rose in relation to the duration of the illness of the person for whom they were caring. Approximately one-quarter were financially affected, and of these, 43 per cent received no financial help of any kind.

'Caring for the Spouse who Died' also contains an important point that is sometimes overlooked: many people who provide lay care are often themselves old, infirm, or in poor health. Indeed, one aspect of the demographic changes mentioned earlier is that, not only are the spouses of people receiving lay care often elderly, so too may be their daughters and sons.

Lay and formal care

So far we have concentrated on describing lay health care in contemporary Britain — what it includes, how much of it there is, and who does it. But we have already noted that lay care and formal care do not exist independently of each other: each affects the other in a variety of ways.

☐ In 'Caring for the Spouse who Died', some of the lay carers mentioned contacts with formal health services. What attitudes did they express about GPs, and about help from nurses?

■ Most of the sample (around 90 per cent) thought the care they had received from GPs was either very good or good. But some of the spouses commented on the inadequate formal nursing help they received, and in one of the reported instances nurses often asked a lay carer (a daughter) to take over from them because they were in a rush: the availability of lay care influenced the formal care offered.

*Bowling, Ann and Cartwright, Ann, 'Caring for the Spouse who Died' in Black, N., et al., ibid.

Relations between lay and formal care are complex, varied, and embrace a wide range of views and opinions. Consider, first, some views of lay health care by the medical profession and others.

In a recent review of lay health manuals, the American doctor John Stoeckle (1984) cites one manual entitled *What You should know about Medical Lab Tests, a complete Guide to understanding all those Tests your Doctor ordered and what the Results mean*. He points out the assumption behind it: that the doctor has too little time to explain properly about laboratory tests, while the reader needs to know about them to become a good patient. In the same vein The Royal Commission on Medical Education (1968) was quite clear as to the goal of lay health education:

> the typical patient of the future — who will be better educated and better informed about health dangers — can be expected to take more responsibility for the management of trivial and self-limiting complaints, provided he is given the necessary encouragement and guidance by the medical profession. (Cited in OHE, 1968, p.26)

This view of lay health care — that it must be guided and informed by *experts* — has led to many schemes for its reordering.

□   What historical examples occur to you?
■   One example cited earlier is the development, following the Boer War, of a system of health visiting; a system designed in part to remodel lay health practices in ways appropriate to a *national* interest.

A good deal of official health education is also based on this view.

We shall illustrate this approach, however, with just one detailed example.

We mentioned earlier (page 86) the way in which health care might be seen as an 'iceberg', with its major part — the lay sector — lying submerged and largely invisible to the public gaze. But the iceberg metaphor has also been used in quite another way. According to the Australian doctor, J.M. Last, there was also a '*clinical iceberg*'. On his analysis in 1963, all kinds of serious disease which only professionals could treat, lay submerged in the lay sector, beyond the view of medical practitioners. The key task of modern formal health services was therefore to reach out into the community, to detect and to treat the formidable burden of disease which had hitherto escaped professional care. Table 6.2 reveals the extent of the problem as Last saw it.

□   What information about formal care would you want before deciding whether Last's objective was appropriate?
■   You would want to know if people with these

DOMESTIC MEDICINE;

OR, THE

FAMILY PHYSICIAN:

BEING AN ATTEMPT

To render the MEDICAL ART more generally useful, by shewing people what is in their own power both with respect to the PREVENTION and CURE of Diseases.

CHIEFLY

Calculated to recommend a proper attention to REGIMEN and SIMPLE MEDICINES.

BY

WILLIAM BUCHAN, M.D.

Sed valitudo fuftentatur notitia fui corporis ; et obferva-tione, quae res aut prodeffe foleant, aut obeffe ; et conti-nentia in victu omni atque cultu, corporis tuendi caufa ; et praetermittendis voluptatibus ; poftremo, arte eorum quorum ad fcientiam haec pertinent. CIC. DE OFFIC.

EDINBURGH:
Printed by BALFOUR, AULD, and SMELLIE.
†
M,DCC,LXIX.

Figure 6.3 Title-page of William Buchan's *Domestic Medicine*, published in Edinburgh in 1769. The book was translated into seven languages and was on sale in the USA until 1913. Buchan was buried in Westminster Abbey.

conditions would benefit from having them detected and treated.

In practice, and partly with the benefit of hindsight, the case for the 'clinical iceberg' is weaker than Last suggested. Several of the conditions he identified and labelled as diseases are in fact only variations of the normal healthy state. For example, a low level of haemoglobin is not synonymous with anaemia needing treatment. The 'iceberg' also includes conditions for which there is no

Table 6.2 The 'clinical iceberg': the experience of one year in a general practice with 2 250 patients — the average number in 1960

Cases of disease recognised by GP		Total number of cases in practice including undetected and potential cases	
Pulmonary TB	6–7	X-ray evidence of TB	12–14
Cervical cancer	0.22	Pre-cancerous lesions	2–3
Anaemia in women aged 15–44	12	Haemoglobin less than 12g per 100ml	114
Diabetes mellitus	14	Sugar in urine	29
Hypertension in men aged over 45	8	Diastolic blood pressure of 100mm of mercury or more in men aged 45 years and above	30
Psychiatric disorders in men aged over 15	27	Conspicuous psychiatric morbidity — males aged over 15	58

(Source: J. M. Last, 1963, p.28)

effective medical treatment, such as minor mental illness, and conditions such as rectal cancer that a doctor could not easily detect without subjecting everyone to regular, expensive and sometimes unpleasant tests and examinations. Finally, Last did not consider the extent to which people with some of these conditions were satisfied with lay treatments. In short, the concept of the 'clinical iceberg' did not sustain a very convincing argument for 'leaving it to the experts'.

One strand running through the concept of the 'clinical iceberg' was the view that lay care was ineffective: that formally untreated disease *should* be formally treated because formal treatment was more effective than lay treatment. There have been other attempts to tackle this question of effectiveness — for instance, by comparing professional and lay views on hypothetical problems that patients might have. Or one could get doctors to evaluate lay treatments which their patients have actually used. Data from a study which used the first method are cited in Table 6.3.

Table 6.3 Comparison of doctors' and lay people's views on self-treatment

Condition	Percentage thinking that self-treatment without consultation is appropriate	
	Doctors	Lay people
Constant depression for 3 weeks	9	26
Difficulty in sleeping for 1 week	58	45
Heavy cold with a temperature and a running nose	86	70
A sore throat for 3 days and nothing else	27	55
Boil that is present after 1 week	12	22
Headache more than once a week for 1 month	17	40

(Source: Dunnell and Cartwright, 1972, Table 40, p.65)

☐ Comment briefly on the differences between the doctors' views and those of lay people.

■ With only two exceptions a lower proportion of doctors — in some cases much lower — considered self-treatment to be appropriate. The two exceptions were sleeping difficulties (where 58 per cent of the doctors favoured self-treatment compared to 45 per cent of lay people) and a heavy cold (for which 86 per cent of doctors considered self-treatment appropriate).

Even where a majority of doctors would favour self-treatment, there is still a significant minority in most cases who would oppose it. At least part of the explanation for this may be a belief amongst doctors that self-treatment is potentially hazardous. In this context it is interesting to look at the very limited information that is available on how doctors evaluate actual lay treatment. A Danish and a British study have both produced very similar results. In the former, a Danish general practitioner concluded that 90 per cent of the lay treatments used by his patients were relevant to their condition, though a third might have only an 'indifferent' effect. The British study involved a panel of doctors working in ten general practices in London. They concluded that two-thirds of the patients who treated themselves used fully or at least partially effective remedies, and only five per cent of the treatments were felt to be even potentially hazardous.

In short, while there is some evidence for the view that the laity are ignorant of some key signs of serious and treatable disease and therefore perhaps need better instruction and investigation, there is also evidence that there is less relevant submerged disease than was once thought, that some doctors are very prone to underestimate the effectiveness of lay diagnosis and treatment, and, not surprisingly perhaps, that experts are liable to overestimate the importance of their special expertise.

Thus, in contrast to the view that lay care calls for aid, supervision and control by experts, it has often been argued that individual patients cannot, need not and should not rely on the state, the medical profession, other experts or indeed anyone else but themselves. From this point of view medical knowledge should be made as freely available as possible, people should treat themselves wherever they can, and formal medical services should play only an ancillary role — doctors and the like are to occupy a strictly subordinate position, giving advice only when asked to do so. Here, it is the patient who is the expert and, indeed, it is seen as every citizen's right, as well as duty, to become expert.

☐ What historical examples of this occur to you?
■ There have been many statements of this point of view: this was Culpeper's aim in publishing his *Herbal*; St Just wished to abolish hospitals and professions; the Thompsonian movement in nineteenth-century America (see Figure 6.3).

In the contemporary world many books and manuals can be found which, like Culpeper's *Herbal*, attempt to give people medical and health care information and advice: to create, if not a populace of experts, at least a populace of well-informed lay people. One of the best-known is *Our Bodies, Ourselves: A Health Book By and For Women*, which was originally published in the USA in 1971 and was subsequently reprinted in Britain and other countries. As the initial authors of that book stated,

we had all experienced frustration and anger towards specific doctors and the medical maze in general, and initially we wanted to do something about this. As we talked we began to realise how little we knew about our own bodies, so we decided to do further research, to prepare papers in groups and then to discuss our findings together. We learned both from professional sources (medical textbooks, journals, doctors, nurses), and from our own experience ... Knowledge has freed us to an extent. It has freed us, for example, from playing the role of mother if it is not a role that fits us. It has given us room to discover the energy and talents that are in us. We want to help make this freedom available to every woman. This is why people in the women's movement have been so active in fighting legal restrictions, the imperfections of available contraceptives, poor sex education, and poorly administered health care that keeps too many women from having this crucial control over their bodies. (Phillips and Rakusen, 1979 edition, pp.11–12)

☐ Contrast this view with that in the quotation cited earlier from the Royal Commission on Medical Education (page 88).
■ The Royal Commission sees the 'typical patient' as having responsibility just for 'trivial and self-limiting complaints' and only then in special circumstances,

'provided he is given the necessary encouragement and guidance by the medical profession'. The patient on this model is weak, ignorant, lacking in confidence and male. In *Our Bodies, Ourselves*, the 'patient' is first and foremost a person, and the issue is not just about 'trivial and self-limiting complaints' but about personal knowledge, freedom and rights.

There are many variants of the view that people should and could take more responsibility for their health. Some are a matter of individual action, such as altering one's diet, or taking more exercise, or giving up health-damaging habits such as smoking; others stress the need for collective action, to accomplish these same goals by forcing change on the food or tobacco or advertising industries, or to attain much wider goals. Virchow's conclusion to his report on the typhus epidemic in Upper Silesia was a good illustration of the latter view (see p.42), urging the need for people to transform their lives by transforming their society.

Conclusion

For all the interest, present and past, in making expertise in health care more available to a wider lay population, there has been an obvious and massive growth in the technical knowledge available to formal health care workers, as well as a major increase in occupations such as health visitors and health education officers. But just as industrial society has aided the growth and power of formal care, so too has it aided some aspects at least of the informal sector. Mass education and mass political organisation, the production of cheap and reliable handbooks, the massive expansion of proprietary medicine and the future possibilities of home-computer diagnosis: all these have strengthened the potential resources open to the lay sector. What conclusions, therefore, can be drawn about lay care and about its relationship with formal care?

We shall close by considering just one set of comparative data — a contrast between the use of pharmaceutical products in towns in the UK, Yugoslavia and the USA.

☐ Examine Figure 6.4. What seems, on this evidence at least, to be the relationship between the extent of self-medication and the volume of drugs formally prescribed by doctors?
■ The rates for both seem to run in parallel. Yugoslavia has both a low prescribing rate and a low self-medication rate. In the UK rates for both are much higher and they are higher still in the USA.
☐ What might account for this?
■ There are several possibilities. The state might be regulating both the lay and professional sectors in the same fashion; or doctors might be setting a fashion for medication which is paralleled in the lay sector; both

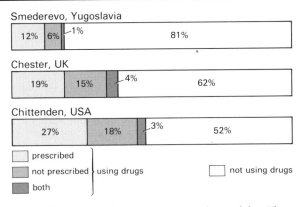

Figure 6.4 Drugs taken in previous two days, adults. Three selected countries
(Source: OHE, 1968, p.12)

sectors might reflect a wider public opinion, or levels of national wealth; or, finally, both might be shaped by the relative power of the pharmaceutical industry.

Whatever the truth of the matter — and things are complicated by the fact that what counts as a prescribed or non-prescribed drug differs in these countries — it is none the less clear that the nature of the lay care sector may differ in certain important respects in different countries. Moreover, it also appears that neither the lay nor the formal sector can be fully understood on their own; each influences the other, and both in turn are shaped by wider social, political and economic forces. But whatever the differences in lay care between countries, and whatever the factors influencing lay and formal care, it seems clear that any account of health care that confines itself to *formal* health care thereby omits most of the health care activity taking place in any society.

Objectives for Chapter 6

When you have studied this chapter, you should be able to:

6.1 Describe the part played by lay care in diagnosis, treatment, personal health maintenance and nursing care.

6.2 Discuss the central role that women play in the main areas of lay health care.

6.3 Outline different views of the relationship between lay and formal health care.

Questions for Chapter 6

1 (*Objective 6.1*)

Where our people have been able to obtain their own medicines and have read books about hygiene or have had relatives, neighbours or travellers to suggest remedies they have been ready in large numbers to rely on such sources and on their own judgements rather than to resort to physicians even with serious ailments. (Cassedy, 1977, p.674)

(i) This statement was written by a contemporary American author. Is it true of contemporary Britain?

(ii) What key aspect of lay care is not mentioned in the above quotation?

2 (*Objective 6.2*)

All the work tends to converge at the same conclusion namely that there are many fairly dependent people being maintained in the community at costs below those of either residential care or long-stay hospital care. (Wright, Cairns and Snell, 1981, p.39)

Why might lay care be cheaper?

3 (*Objective 6.3*) A distinction was made earlier in the text between the 'iceberg' of health care (in which only the formal part appears in public view) and the 'clinical iceberg' of disease.

Why might doctors tend to stress the notion of the 'clinical iceberg', and why might the notion of the 'iceberg' of health care be emphasised by people opposed to a monopoly of expertise?

7

Empires and exchanges: a world health care system?

We began this book by stressing the need to adopt a historical *and* a comparative perspective on health care. The ideal would be to sustain both perspectives simultaneously, but beginning with the broad canvas of the Mediterranean world of antiquity, with European-wide developments in health care, and with early exchanges between Europe and the rest of the world, successive chapters have been obliged to narrow the focus: Europe alone, then north-west Europe, and finally Britain and indeed England have come to the fore.

This has happened for a number of reasons. First, practical constraints of time and space have made it necessary to illustrate by means of detailed example the sheer range of activities that caring for health embraces, and the wide range of influences that social life exerts on health care. No one country's health care history is identical to any other's, but this range of activities and of influences is a basic lesson that any country's health care history would afford. And the history of health care in Britain is typical in the sense that it can only be understood by looking beyond national boundaries: it is less a national history than a history of events, circumstances, influences and ideas into which the history of health care fits in a particular way.

☐ What aspects of European history, for example, have fundamentally altered British health care?

■ Among the most important examples are the Roman occupation, the Europe-wide organisation of the Church, the revival of Greek learning in the Italian city-states, the Leyden hospital, the French Revolution and the reorganisation of medical practice, the introduction of health insurance in Germany, and the Crimean and twentieth-century wars.

Second, there are *historiographical* reasons for narrowing the focus; that is, reasons to do with the writing of history and the data that are available. The craft of the historian is essentially a European invention, and it is a craft that is practised in different languages: an immensely powerful bias exists towards concentrating on that fraction of recorded history that is written in one's native language.

The third reason is rather different. For most of the period covered in earlier chapters, it would not be too wild a generalisation to state that European — or British — health care was not decisively different from health care or medicine in other parts of the world. Chinese, Indian, or Islamic health care and medical knowledge may have held no all-round advantage in sophistication, effectiveness, scientific theory or technique, but until quite recently they were ahead in some areas and were certainly at no overall disadvantage. But, as we noted at the end of Chapter 2, this approximate equality broke down. By the end of the fifteenth century Europe had embarked on a long epoch of world-wide expansion, trading, migrating, colonising and changing the rest of the world. For a while, Britain was at the very heart of this global expansion. Hence, a crucial reason exists for pursuing the history of health care in Europe and more particularly in Britain from the late fifteenth century onwards; health care in the rest of the world would also be changed by British and European developments and would have to come to terms with them.

So this book has now reached the stage where it is possible once again to broaden the canvas, to begin to consider the impact that the 'Age of Europe' has had on the rest of the world's health care, and to look more systematically at the diversity of health care in the contemporary world. We start by sketching briefly some of the encounters between Europe and other parts of the world after 1500, then look in more detail at one aspect of the contemporary world that in some ways typifies the 'global village' of health care: the migration of health care workers around the world.

The global spread of European health care

The global spread of European health care was just one aspect of the massive expansion in European influence from the sixteenth century onwards. The Portuguese initially set the pace, establishing a trading post at Goa on the west coast of India in 1510, and by the mid-sixteenth century had founded a series of fortified towns from Angola in southern Africa to Zanzibar in east Africa. From India they progressed to Macao in China via Malacca in the Malay archipelago. Meanwhile the Spanish went west, to Mexico, Panama, Peru, and Chile.

Europeans altered patterns of health care in several ways in the territories they were beginning to acquire. First, they took with them their own medical knowledge and health care practices; second, they destroyed or modified existing indigenous health care in the territories they colonised; third, they spread European diseases to those territories;* and fourth, partly as a consequence of suffering from unfamiliar diseases, the Europeans sought ways of combating the diseases of the tropics and the New World. However, the flow of ideas and knowledge was not entirely one way. Europeans assimilated into their own system some of the drugs, techniques, procedures and knowledge of indigenous systems that they encountered in almost every corner of the world.

By the mid-sixteenth century the Spanish were the only Europeans who had moved to their colonies in any numbers

— around 120 000 had moved to the Americas by 1560. The main British colony was in North America, to which around 50 000 people had moved by 1660. In the eighteenth century this movement of peoples began to swell rapidly: around 200 000 Portuguese moved to Brazil, 250 000 Germans moved to America, and no fewer than 2.5 million British and Dutch to North America. In the nineteenth century migration expanded even more (Table 7.1).

As André Armengaud, an economic historian, has commented:

> Taken as a whole European emigration probably represents the greatest transfer of populations in the history of mankind ... never before had one continent exercised so great an influence on the rest.
> (Armengaud, 1976, pp.70, 72)

Let us look at the various effects that this had on health care. First, the Europeans took with them their own forms of health care. Thus, having set up a trading post in India in 1608, the British East India Company opened their first hospital for Europeans (in Madras) in 1664; their first hospital for Indian soldiers did not open until 1760 and the first for civilians until 1792. Where some provision was made for civilians, the priority groups were usually those employed in European-owned mines, plantations, and factories. This can be seen in Ghana, where mine and harbour installations were provided with hospitals for the African labour force. The often highly restricted coverage of such services is indicated by the fact that a meagre 0.02 per cent of the Ghanian population had access to these hospital services in the early twentieth century.

But in other cases health care services were more broadly cast. In 1839 the British government sanctioned a system to counter smallpox in the West Indian colonies:

Table 7.1 Migration of Europeans in the nineteenth century

Period	From	To	Number
1821–1910	Scandinavia	USA	1.7 million
1821–1910	Ireland	USA	4.1 million
1821–1910	Germany	USA	5 million
1821–1910	UK	USA and British colonies	12.7 million
1821–1910	France	North Africa	1.5 million
1821–1910	Europe	South America	3.6 million
1890–1910	USSR	USA	2 million
1900–1910	Italy	USA	2 million

(Sources: *The Times Atlas of World History*, 1984, pp.208–9, and Armengaud, 1976, pp.60–72)

*This effect of European expansion is discussed in more detail in *Medical Knowledge: Doubt and Certainty* and *The Health of Nations, ibid*. (U205 Books II and III).

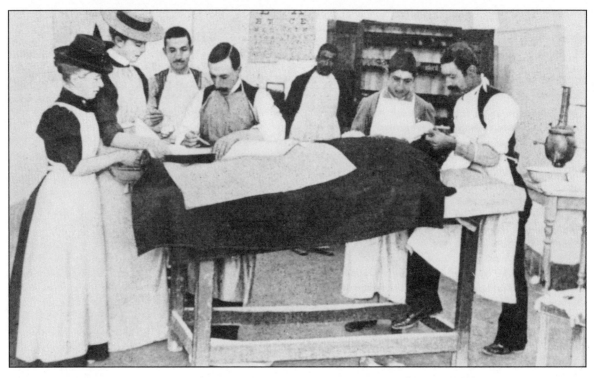

Figure 7.1 An operation in progress at the Church Missionary Society's Hospital at Yezd, Persia, around 1890.

The Barbadoes Board of Health in 1839 offered free vaccination to all who insisted ... Vaccinators General were established, who were to visit all houses of all classes on the island and vaccinate everyone living there. (Hodgkinson, 1967, p.129)

□ How did such measures compare with those in Britain at the time?

■ They went considerably beyond those sanctioned by the Poor Law.

In the early phases, the spread of European health care was propelled by commercial and military superiority rather than by any advantage in medical effectiveness. One contemporary account of the efficacy of an East India Company hospital in 1708 paints a general picture rather succinctly:

The Company has a pretty good hospital at Calcutta, where many go in to undergo the Penance of Physic, but few come out to give an account of its operation. (Cited in McDonald, 1950, p.85)

Apart from exporting health services to the newly acquired colonies, the European powers also established medical training. For example, the first medical school in America, opened in 1765 in Philadelphia, was staffed entirely by

graduates from Edinburgh. Indeed, the Edinburgh medical school's records are a good illustration of this process of diffusion: graduates established medical schools in Bombay and Calcutta (India), in Otago (New Zealand), in Sydney (Australia), in Lima (Peru), in Dalhousie and Kingston, Ontario (Canada). Nor were such influences limited to medical buildings. The social security systems in Latin America, that later had a strong influence on national health policies, were often introduced by Europeans. For example, mutual benefit societies providing hospital care were introduced to Cuba by Spanish settlers.

Quite apart from the activities of the formal administrations, *missionaries* were active in health care in many colonies. Some missionary organisations had existed from an early date: the Society for Promoting Christian Knowledge was founded in 1698, the Society for the Propagation of the Gospel in 1701, both with the initial intention of converting 'heathens' to Christianity. However, by the nineteenth century, many such societies had developed an orientation to health work. In China, medical missionaries from the west had been arriving since the 1830s. From travelling practices, these missionaries gradually established clinics, then hospitals, and finally medical colleges and teaching schools. In parts of China, missions organised rural medical services that in some respects prefigured the 'barefoot' health workers of the 1960s.

Although the tendency in the nineteenth century was for European health care to supplant indigenous systems, interest had been shown in the latter during earlier centuries. First, many of the diseases that the Europeans encountered were completely new to them, and they had no knowledge or experience of how to respond to them. Second, the first colonists often arrived without any European physicians or remedies, and were sometimes forced to rely on indigenous skills.

Thus the sixteenth-century Spanish *conquistadores* had been obliged to employ Aztec physicians to tend their sick and wounded. Cortez was apparently sufficiently impressed with their skills to despatch a letter to the Spanish King informing him that there was no need to send Spanish physicians to the New World. Later, in 1570, Philip II of Spain did despatch his personal physician Francisco Hernandez to Mexico, but to gather systematic information on Aztec medicines, a task that Hernandez took seven years to accomplish. Many plants and herbs were imported to Europe by all colonial powers. The Physick Garden in Oxford, which opened in 1632 had, within twenty years, accumulated 1 000 'exotics', compared to the 600 native plants. By 1661 the Royal Society had set up a committee to collect information on all aspects of the 'medical topography of distant lands'.

The most famous example of medicine imported from the New World was a remedy for the much-dreaded malaria. In the seventeenth century Europeans in Peru learnt of the indigenous medical practice of using the powdered bark of a native tree referred to by Peruvians as *quina-quina* ('bark of bark'). The use of this powder spread rapidly to Europe and was disseminated widely by Europeans to other parts of the world. Jesuit missionaries played a role in the spread of the bark's use, and it was known for a while as 'Jesuit's bark'. It has been claimed that French Jesuits in China used the bark to cure the Chinese Emperor Sheng-Tsu of malaria. If true, it is an early example of the medical 'global village'. In 1822 the active principle of this bark was isolated by two French chemists, and named 'quinine'.

In India, too, Europeans were:

> ... keen to learn as much as they could from local practitioners and their knowledge of indigenous drugs ... they studied and catalogued the local medicinal plants. John Marshall, a trader in Bengal from 1668 to 1677, described the systems of Hindu science and medicine that he had learned from local practitioners. He and his contemporaries often tried the local remedies, and proved their efficacy ... The European surgeons slowly learned to modify their heroic

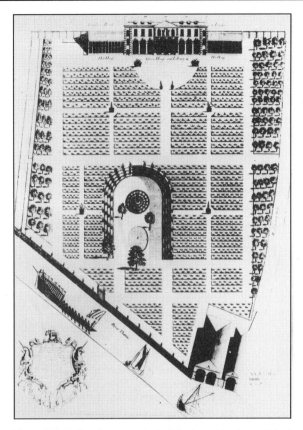

Figure 7.2 Medieval monasteries kept herb gardens for medicinal purposes, but the seventeenth century saw an explosive growth of physic gardens, well stocked with exotics. The spirit of rationalism is evident in this engraving of the layout of the Physick Garden in Chelsea. The stock has been maintained and the garden is now open to the public.

> methods of treatment that they had brought with them (bleeding, purging, and the excessive use of mercury). They soon noticed that Indians were relatively immune to some of the local diseases, and there were attempts to increase the resistance of Europeans by the process of 'indianization' (bleeding or starving followed by a diet exclusively of Indian food) to make their blood more like that of the Indians ... (Patterson, 1983, p.465)

At the end of the eighteenth century Europeans were enthusiastically taking up the skills of Indian surgical work in the area of rhinoplasty (repairing the nasal bones). Indeed plastic surgery's evolution can be traced directly to this source.

European interest in indigenous care seems to have come to an end in the nineteenth century. Increasingly, European health care supplanted, and sometimes destroyed, existing systems. In India, the British closed down all the colleges teaching indigenous systems in 1833. Later, between 1912 and 1917, a series of Acts made it illegal for a registered practitioner to be associated with Indian medicine. In China, events followed a similar course. In 1929 the Kuomintang government initiated a series of measures greatly to reduce the use of Chinese medicine and stimulate the spread of western practices: these included the banning of schools of traditional medicine and of the publication of books and articles on the subject. Likewise in Thailand, the royal court increasingly accepted European medicine from the late nineteenth century onwards, and in 1892 the first 'modern' medical school was opened, though this taught Thai as well as European medicine. But by 1907 the latter had supplanted the indigenous system — at least with regard to health care for the growing urban élite. What is striking about such events is the rapidity with which countries adopted the European system. This was true of Japan. Although the Japanese had had some contact with western medicine in the late eighteenth century, this virtually ceased until they reopened their country to westerners in 1854. By 1883 only doctors who had studied western medicine were granted licences to practise.

A further effect on health care of European expansion was the interest it produced in Europeans about the diseases of the tropics and the New World. It rapidly became apparent that successful colonisation was going to require the means of overcoming the diseases peculiar to these areas. Even in North America most of the very earliest white settlers died within two years of arrival. And in Africa, Asia and South America, disease presented an even greater obstacle to expansion. For example, in 1765 the French had attempted to establish a colony in Guinea in West Africa: 80 per cent of the 10 000 colonists who went were dead within months of arrival. It is a striking fact that more French colonial settlers left for Guinea than for Canada. The latter, however, was not such a 'white man's grave', and the immigrants consequently thrived.

European expeditions were continually hampered by disease: in the 1816 Congo expedition, twenty-one dead out of forty-four; in the Niger expedition of 1832 there were thirty-two dead out of forty-one. The expedition to the Gambia in 1805 led by Mungo Park, a botanist and graduate of Edinburgh medical school, was a particularly dramatic case in point:

> Your Lordship will recollect that I always spoke of the rainy season with horror, as being extremely fatal to Europeans; and our journey from the Gambia to the Niger will furnish a melancholy proof of it. We had no contact with the natives, nor was any one of us killed by wild animals or any other accidents; and yet I am sorry to say that of forty-four Europeans

> who left the Gambia in perfect health five only are at the present alive — viz., three soldiers (one deranged in his mind), lieutenant Maclyn and myself. (Park, cited in Basch, 1978, p.60)

It was obstacles such as these that acted as a spur to investigating and understanding how these diseases were transmitted. In 1877 Patrick Manson, an Aberdeen graduate working in Hong Kong, demarcated the role of the mosquito in transmitting malaria. His findings met with an incredulous response, but further evidence from others, including Alphonse Laveran, a French army officer in Algeria, and Ronald Ross, an army doctor in India, confirmed Manson's findings. At almost the same time, it was established that mosquitoes also played a key role in the transmission of yellow fever, and that the tsetse fly was responsible for the transmission of sleeping sickness (trypanosomiasis) in Africa. In the space of a very few years, therefore, it was discovered by Europeans working in colonial territories that insects played a key role in transmitting three of the worst disease hazards in the colonies. The opportunity to demonstrate the value of this knowledge came in Panama in central America at the beginning of the twentieth century.

In 1880, Ferdinand de Lesseps, a French engineer famous for his construction of the Suez Canal, had begun work on a canal project in Panama. Between 1880 and 1888, as a result of endemic malaria and yellow fever, the company lost 20 000 workers and 300 million dollars, went bankrupt and abandoned the project. Around 1900, it was demonstrated in Cuba, then an American colony, that yellow fever could be controlled by attacking the mosquitoes' breeding grounds. Construction on the canal recommenced:

> By 1905 more than 400 men were employed in mosquito extermination alone ... Piped water supplies were constructed to eliminate the barrels that had formerly produced clouds of mosquitoes. Houses were screened and bed-nets provided for the canal workers. Quinine was issued both as a prophylactic against malaria and a cure, and persons with fevers were isolated behind screening. (Basch, 1978, p.66)

By the completion date of the canal — 1914 — the death rate in the Panama zone had fallen from 176 to 6 per thousand.

As noted earlier, it was not obvious up to the nineteenth century that European health care had any decisive advantage over other systems. But the application of the scientific method to insect-borne diseases gave the European system a clear advantage. Here was a demonstration that in the case of at least some diseases it worked better than any alternative.

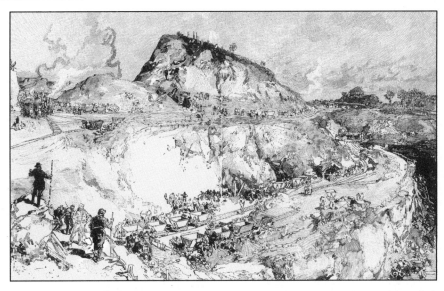

Figure 7.3 Panama in 1884, midway through de Lesseps' doomed project. But when work restarted, 'as the engineers blasted and dredged, the war waged against *Aedes* and *Anopheles* by the sanitarians gradually brought yellow fever and malaria under control and marked a high point in the history of applied epidemiology . . .' (Basch, 1978, p.66).

☐ In what other main area had western medicine secured a decisive advantage by the end of the nineteenth century?

■ Surgery, using aseptic procedures.

It was these two factors — the study of infectious disease and the new techniques of surgery — that convinced many in non-European countries that their indigenous systems of health care were in need of serious modification. There were, however, still to be many points of friction between the old and new systems.

Contemporary health care: an international trade

In 1945, there were around fifty recognised independent countries — forty of which were in Europe or the Americas: much of the world was still in the colonial possession of European powers. By 1984, liberation movements and colonial withdrawal had increased the number of independent nation-states to around 160, over half of which were in Africa and Asia. As you have already seen, however, national borders are porous to the movement of people, materials and ideas, and it is these movements that represent the essence of what is meant here by international health care.

☐ Can you suggest some ways in which international exchanges take place?

■ There are many, but four of the main ones are: the migration of health workers, in particular doctors and nurses; the movement of ideas and knowledge via journals, books and conferences; the provision of health services by international agencies such as the World Health Organization (WHO); and the trade in drugs and medical equipment.

Before looking in more detail at one specific aspect of these exchanges — migration — let's briefly note the following points. First, the scale of the international pharmaceutical trade is enormous. In 1980 total world consumption of pharmaceutical products amounted to almost $80 000 million. Second, western companies dominate this trade. Although about 10 000 companies were producing these products, about 100 producers accounted for almost 90 per cent of total production, and a mere twenty-five of these manufactured 44 per cent of it. Of these twenty-five largest pharmaceutical companies in the world, four are German, three Swiss, thirteen American, one French, one Japanese and three British (Glaxo at number twenty, Beecham, twenty-three, and ICI, twenty-five). These companies effectively control world production, while most Third World countries produce few or no pharmaceutical products at all. Forty-five of the poorest and smallest countries are entirely dependent on imported drugs. Multinational companies also take a large share of the market in larger countries such as India (70 per cent foreign share), Argentina (59 per cent) and Brazil (88 per cent). Taken as a whole, the net import bill for pharmaceuticals from the industrialised countries to Third World countries was $4 000 million in 1980, and although this represented

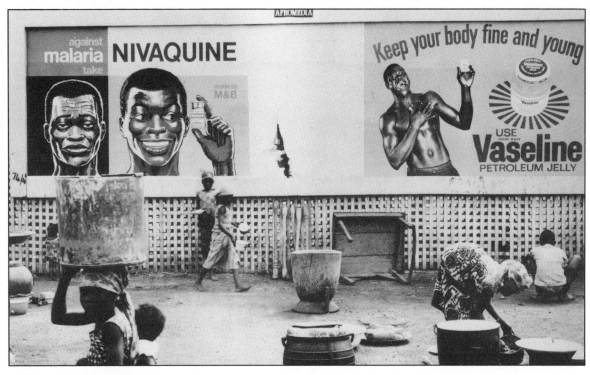

Figure 7.4 Third World advertising. In 1980 the international pharmaceutical industry allocated one per cent of total research and development spending to specifically Third-World drug research. Some companies, such as Wellcome and May and Baker (manufacturers of Nivaquine) do more in this respect than others.

only some 2 per cent of their total imports, it has also been one of the most rapidly growing items.*

However, there are a number of countries that have developed policies to control and plan their use of pharmaceuticals. Some, such as India, China, Egypt, Cuba and Bangladesh have acted to reduce import dependence by setting up their own state-run drug manufacturing plants. Others have tried to regulate the drugs they import. In Sri Lanka, for example, following a government-sponsored review of the 4 000 drugs in use in 1962, a list of 600 approved or essential drugs was drawn up and import licences withdrawn from the remainder. In Mozambique the same process cut the list of routinely supplied drugs from 13 000 to 355.

In drawing up policies like these, some countries have been able to draw on technical assistance from international agencies such as the WHO. The first attempts to create an international health organisation all focused on infectious diseases and discussions of quarantine regulations. In 1851 an International Sanitary Conference was held in Paris, in the wake of the cholera pandemics of 1828–1831 and 1847. One of the first international health conventions to be agreed, in 1892, was confined to monitoring and regulating the movement of pilgrims to and from Mecca. (The Mecca pilgrimage was thought to have spread cholera throughout Islamic areas of the world.) The development of more broadly based international health cooperation was accelerated with the formation of a Health Organization in 1923 attached to the League of Nations. It was through the Health Organization that Greek public health was reorganised in 1928, that China in 1929 received technical aid, that Poland and Romania mounted a programme to control typhus.

The Health Organization formed the foundations of the WHO, created in 1946 as an agency of the United Nations to promote international cooperation in the field of health care. The WHO has been closely identified with programmes based on so-called 'search and destroy' tactics, that is, trying to find effective technical laboratory-based solutions to specific health problems. While the WHO is the largest single intergovernmental organisation involved in health care, there are many others including the UN International Children's Emergency Fund (UNICEF) and the Food and Agriculture Organization (FAO). In

*Further aspects of the pharmaceutical industry are considered in *Caring for Health: Dilemmas and Prospects, ibid.* (U205 Book VII).

addition, voluntary organisations such as Save the Children Fund, Oxfam and War on Want operate on an international scale.

These briefly considered aspects of international exchange suggest that there exists something that might be called a world health care system. In order to gain some idea of the wide-ranging factors involved in such exchanges the rest of this chapter is devoted to a more detailed discussion of the international movement of nurses and doctors, a topic that at times has attracted considerable interest and controversy.

In 1972 migrant doctors constituted two groups: around 5 000 temporary migrants working on various technical aid projects, and 140 000 (equivalent to 6 per cent of the world total) who had moved permanently from the country where they were born or were trained. Although 6 per cent does not sound a particularly large number, most had moved to a very small number of recipient countries: 119 000 (86 per cent) were to be found in either the USA (77 000), the United Kingdom (21 000), Canada (11 000), West Germany (6 000) or Australia (4 000). Putting these figures another way, 25 per cent of all doctors in the USA were foreign medical graduates, 25 per cent in the UK, and 33 per cent in Canada.

☐   Is the migration of doctors a recent phenomenon?
■   No, as you have seen, Greek physicians migrated throughout the city-states that made up the Hellenistic world, and in medieval times physicians from Salerno migrated throughout Europe.

Which countries do doctors emigrate from today? Here things get a bit more complicated, because some countries that are recipients of foreign medical graduates are also donors. For instance, in 1972 there were 21 000 doctors who had moved to the UK and 8 000 who had emigrated from it. The main donor countries, however, are India, with around 15 000 doctors working abroad, and the Philippines, with around 10 000.

Less is known about the migration of nurses, but in the 1970s around 15 000 were estimated to move each year, which would suggest that around 6 per cent of all the world's nurses are working somewhere other than their country of birth or training. And, as with doctors, most migrating nurses go to a very small number of countries: 90 per cent to just eight countries, chiefly the USA, UK and Canada. The nurses moving around the world each year come from a much more scattered range of countries, but the main exporters in 1972 were the Philippines (2 400), the UK (2 000) and Australia (1 500).

If the world is divided into industrialised countries and Third World countries, the picture that emerges is as follows: 44 per cent of migrant doctors came from an industrialised country, and 56 per cent from a Third World country, while 89 per cent went to an industrialised country and 11 per cent to a Third World country. For nurses the pattern is similar: 60 per cent came from an industrialised country and 40 per cent from a Third World country, while 94 per cent went to an industrialised country and only 6 per cent to a Third World country.

☐   How would you summarise the broad pattern of these flows of health workers in terms of the relative wealth of the countries involved?
■   The general direction of migration is from poorer countries to richer countries.

These figures on the size and direction of migration among doctors and nurses give rise to two questions: why does migration occur, and what are the consequences for the countries involved?

☐   What possible reasons are there for migration?
■   To find employment, to get more pay, and to obtain training and experience are the main reasons.

A WHO study in 1979 concluded that the reasons for migration could be divided into two broad categories: factors that tended to *push* health workers out of donor countries, and factors tending to *pull* health workers into recipient countries. Among the push-factors, the fundamental one was that some countries train more doctors and nurses than they can afford to employ. Argentina and Uruguay, for example, having considerably expanded medical training since the 1960s, reached the position where doctors were unable to find medical work in their own country, and were either taking alternative employment — taxi driving, for instance — or migrating. This lack of connection between the number of doctors or nurses a country trains and the number it can afford to employ is compounded by the fact that the type of training is often based on teaching curricula that have been transferred from much richer countries — another feature of the 'global village' of health care that has been created this century.

☐   How might such curricula be inappropriate to the requirements of the countries to which they have been transplanted, and how might they help to encourage migration?
■   First, the pattern of disease is different in poorer countries: a predominance of infectious diseases among children and young adults rather than degenerative diseases among the old. Second, the treatments in use in wealthy countries are often so expensive that poorer countries cannot afford them. In consequence, many doctors and nurses in poorer countries are more appropriately qualified to work in wealthier countries.

On the other side of this equation, the main pull-factor is

that some of the richer countries train an insufficient number of doctors for their needs, and can therefore offer employment opportunities to immigrants. In the 1960s, the lowering of immigration barriers and the granting of employment permits by richer recipient countries brought forth a large increase in the number of doctors and nurses migrating. However, in the late 1970s and early 1980s, immigration barriers were raised again and qualification criteria tightened to reduce the flow. This was because the rich industrialised countries of western Europe and North America were then producing enough, or even too many, of their own doctors. The increase in the output of medical schools in western European countries between 1960 and 1982 is shown in Table 7.2.

Although the exact number of unemployed doctors in western Europe is uncertain, there is no doubt that some countries are dramatically overproducing. In 1983 it was estimated that there were 30 000 unemployed doctors in Italy, and in Belgium there were doctors treating only one or two patients a week!

But why do some countries produce more doctors and nurses than they can afford to employ, while others produce less? In both cases part of the answer seems to lie in the social and economic structure and policies of the countries involved, and the wider social and economic relations between donor and recipient countries. The post-war period saw a rapid increase in employment in richer recipient countries across a whole range of 'service' activities: health, education, welfare, leisure and so on. At the same time, however, some occupations within this broad service sector, such as medicine, were tightly organised into professional groups that had a degree of control over training and qualification: a strategy, as previous chapters have suggested, that helped to raise the status and earnings of the profession by restricting supply. In these circumstances, the relaxation of controls on immigration offered a way of meeting the expanding

demand for doctors and nurses without permanently lowering their status, which might have resulted from a major expansion of domestic output. Migration rates can be adjusted much more rapidly than training rates.

A second attraction of migration from the point of view of recipient countries is that immigrants are more likely to accept low-status jobs than are home-produced staff. The effect of this can be seen in the medical staffing of the NHS, in which 31 per cent of *all* hospital doctors in 1981 had been trained overseas, but only 17 per cent of consultants (the highest grade) had been. Similarly, foreign graduates are over-represented in lower-status specialities such as psychiatry, and under-represented in higher-status specialities such as surgery. Although little research has been carried out on nurse employment, it appears that similar patterns exist.

A frequently expressed view of why some donor countries consistently produce far more doctors and nurses than they can afford to employ is summarised in the concluding sections of the WHO report:

> ... the power-holding élite in the countries concerned largely share the values and tastes of affluent societies and are thus willing partners in the perpetuation of the patterns of production and consumption in those societies. This élite include ... the economic élite; health planners and health administrators; and professional health personnel, e.g. physicians, dentists and health researchers. The decisions made by these groups are based on the needs of that layer of society to which these groups are exposed and whose life-styles induce a pattern of illness that is not representative of the country as a whole but highly resembles that of affluent societies everywhere ...
> (Mejia, *et al.*, 1979, pp.411–12)

Do the patterns of migration described matter, and if so to whom? In trying to assess the consequences of the migration of health workers, let us consider the example of a Malaysian doctor:

A young person of Indian ancestry but born in Malaysia, where he received primary and secondary education at the public expense, decides to study medicine. He goes to Madras, India, for undergraduate medical education and training. His family covers the cost of his tuition and personal expenses during that time. As a part of his clinical training, he provides a certain amount of health services to patients in India. Once he obtains his medical degree, he returns to Malaysia to practise medicine and, after a few years of rendering services in Malaysia with the medical skills he obtained in India, he moves to Canada for training in a medical

Table 7.2 Medical staff, 1960–1982, in western European countries

Country	1960	1982	Increase
Belgium	11 380	26 000	× 2.28
West Germany	79 350	178 000	× 2.24
Denmark	5 525	13 000	× 2.35
France	45 000	143 000	× 3.18
Ireland	3 000	5 000	× 1.66
Italy	80 350	200 000	× 2.50
Luxembourg	319	567	× 1.78
Netherlands	12 800	28 000	× 2.19
United Kingdom	59 600	90 000	× 1.5

(Source: Brearley, 1984, p.1361)

Table 7.3 The effects of health worker migration (1972)

	Ratio per 10 000 population of			
	Doctors		Nurses	
	Actual	Without migration	Actual	Without migration
Industrialised countries	18.1	17.4	32.3	31.8
Third World countries	3.2	3.5	2.7	3.0
World	8.2	8.2	12.7	12.7

(Source: derived from Mejia, *et al.*, 1979, p.170)

speciality. At this point in time he carries with him the primary and secondary education obtained in Malaysia, the undergraduate medical education obtained in India, and the additional medical experience gained in Malaysia. During his speciality training in Canada, which is paid for by the Government of Malaysia, he provides services to patients in Canada. Eventually he migrates to the United States of America with the total of the knowledge and skills obtained — at a cost in terms of both money and time — in three other countries.
(Mejia, *et al.*, 1979, p.148)

What factors need to be taken into account in assessing the losses and gains of each country involved? Table 7.3 shows what would happen to the ratio of health workers in industrialised countries and Third World countries if no migration had occurred, compared with the actual situation.

☐ How would you summarise the actual and hypothetical positions?
■ Industrialised countries are slightly better off and Third World countries slightly worse off than if no migration had occurred, but these differences are insignificant in comparison with the gulf in the overall level of provision between the industrialised and Third World countries. With or without migration the former have between five and ten times as many doctors and nurses per head of population as the latter.
☐ What strikes you as unrealistic about the comparison between the actual position and the hypothetical position?
■ As you saw earlier, a fundamental reason for migration is the lack of employment in donor countries. This would still be the case if every migrant doctor or nurse were to go back to the country they trained in.

Another way of assessing the impact of migration is in terms of the costs to recipient or donor countries of producing or replacing the health workers they gain or lose by migration. For example, if each overseas-trained doctor working in the UK in 1981 had instead been trained in the UK, at a cost of approximately £35 000 per doctor, the total additional cost to the country would have been about £530 million. In the USA, these 'savings' would have amounted to almost six billion dollars in 1973. But again care must be taken in interpreting these figures: first, it cannot be assumed that recipient countries would otherwise have produced the doctors that do migrate to them; second, it is not necessarily the case that a recipient country's gain is the same as a donor country's loss. The cost of training a doctor in the USA was $83 000 in 1973, whereas in Thailand it was $18 000, in the Lebanon $10 000, and in Colombia and Sri Lanka around $5 000. (Although it must be noted that substantial additional costs may be borne by families rather than the state.) Even so, it is evident that recipient countries do gain and donor countries do lose by migration. The loss to donor countries is not so much the loss of a doctor or nurse, but rather the loss of the investment in their training, which could have been used for other purposes. Table 7.4 gives some examples of what might have been done for the cost of training each doctor.

Whether one trained doctor is less 'appropriate' than, for example, nineteen auxiliary sanitarians is a complex question that will be returned to in Chapter 9. And, of course, the question of appropriateness could be asked not

Table 7.4 The relative costs of training health workers

The number of other health workers who could be trained for the cost of educating one doctor in:

Thailand	=	9 nurses or
		19 auxiliary sanitarians
East Africa	=	3 nurses or
		15 auxiliary sanitarians or
		20 medical assistants or
		30 auxiliary nurses
Colombia	=	8 nurses or
		25 auxiliary nurses
Pakistan	=	4 nurses or
		24 medical assistants or
		24 health visitors or
		60 midwives or
		60 sanitary inspectors

(Source: derived from Mejia, *et al.*, 1979, p.149)

only about different types of health workers, but also about pharmaceutical products, hospitals, or many other aspects of health care.

What we have seen, however, is that such questions cannot be posed in isolation from the constant international exchanges, forming what we have referred to as a 'global village' of health care. These exchanges are partly related to the comparative effectiveness of health care, whether this be *quina-quina*, aseptic surgery, or Indian rhinoplasty. But it is clearly not just about effectiveness, it is also about economic strength and weakness, about commerce, custom and culture. Not least, it is about history and how the modern world reflects the past, for many aspects of international health care can be traced to developments discussed earlier in this book, particularly to the gap which opened up between Europe and the rest of the world from around the late fifteenth century. 'To explain this gap, which was to grow wider over the years, is to tackle the essential problem of the history of the modern world' (Braudel, 1982, p.134), and a full explanation must await the rest of the world producing its own history, its own version of events. But as we look more closely at the diversity of health care in the contemporary world, the consequences of this gap form a constant accompaniment.

Objectives for Chapter 7

When you have studied this chapter, you should be able to:

7.1 Describe the consequences both for European and indigenous health care systems of European contact with the tropics, the New World and the Far East up to the twentieth century.

7.2 Explain what is meant by describing modern health care as having become part of a 'global village', and give some examples of how this is manifested.

Questions for Chapter 7

1 (*Objective 7.1*) What was the European attitude to indigenous health care during the seventeenth and eighteenth centuries, and how did this change in the nineteenth century?

2 (*Objective 7.2*) What effect might the opening of a new medical school in the UK have on a newly qualified doctor in India?

8

Formal health care: questions of finance

So far, we have laid great stress on the sheer diversity of health care: the wide range of activities that health care includes, the variety of reasons for providing health care, the many economic, political, religious and other influences upon it. In this chapter we want to take a more systematic look at health care in different countries at the present time, and to try to uncover some recurring patterns within this diversity.

To do this, what is required is a set of questions that can be asked of the health care activities of any society, and a selection of countries that illustrate the full range of possible responses to these questions. By this point in the book, many such questions could be raised. For example, under what circumstances are public health reforms implemented or neglected? What factors influence moves towards or away from institutional confinement? How different are lay care activities from one country to another? What determines the appearance of licensing arrangements for certain health workers? And so on.

The questions asked in this chapter are concentrated on one particular part of health care — formal health services offering mainly personal care. The questions broadly are as follows.

1 What kinds of different organisations are involved in providing these health care services, and how do they raise the money to do so?

2 How much do different countries spend on these health services, and why is there so much variation?

3 What are these health care resources spent on, and how different are the activities of different formal health care systems?

4 What effect does the amount of formal health care provision seem to have on levels of health?

Our choice of this list of questions has not been gratuitous: the fact is that these are the questions that dominate contemporary comparative research on health care, and there is little or no information at present to begin to answer many of the other questions that could be asked. But there is one additional question that might be asked at various points in the chapter: how do the results of this contemporary comparative research on formal health care appear in the light of what we have seen of the full diversity of health care in the book so far?

In asking these questions we have focused on a few countries, so that a basic outline of their formal health care services can gradually be pieced together: they include the USA and USSR, India and China, Japan, Brazil, Ghana, Nicaragua and Britain.

Finance and organisation

In previous chapters we have encountered many different groups of people and organisations involved in the provision of formal health care. An attempt to categorise them has been made by the American epidemiologist, Paul Basch, who came up with the following list.

1 Self-employed indigenous and traditional healers.

2 Private, profit-making health care businesses.

3 Charitable and voluntary organisations.

4 Member-supported non-profit organisations.

5 Privately owned mines, factories, etc., providing health care mainly for their own workers.

6 Government run or supervised health insurance or sickness funds, funded through earmarked contributions.

7 National or local government schemes, funded through taxation. (Basch, 1978, p.273)

In practice, these categories often overlap, and many different categories may simultaneously be involved in a

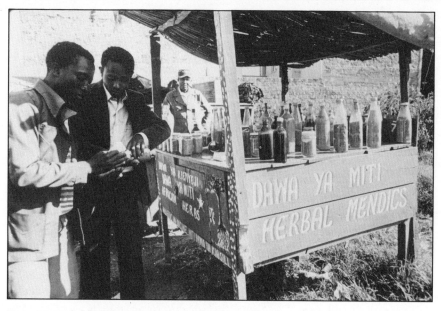

Figure 8.1 Herbal Mendics: a herbal doctor's market stall in Nyeri, Kenya.

country's health care. But let's go through the list and illustrate it with some examples.

Indigenous and traditional healers comprise the bulk of people involved in health care in many countries of the world. India contains around 300 000 people practising indigenous medicine, compared to fewer than 200 000 trained in modern medicine. Similarly in China, the numbers involved in traditional medicines are still greater than doctors trained in modern medicine. These two countries are most often referred to in respect of indigenous health care because some attempts have been made there to integrate these forms of practice with wider health care policies. However, indigenous healers also exist in large numbers in other countries that have no such policies: in Tanzania there are estimated to be upwards of 30 000 traditional practitioners, compared with fewer than 1 200 modern doctors (see Figure 8.1). Traditional healers have been excluded from practice or legally restricted in other countries: in the USSR and Cuba most forms of traditional or 'complementary' medicine are illegal, and in much of Europe the law prohibits most forms of non-registered medical practice. (One instance of this prohibition was a 'dawn swoop' by police on chiropractors in Brussels in 1978.) Despite the legal position it has been estimated that around 5 per cent of the population in most European countries still make regular use of these practitioners. In the UK the total number of 'complementary' therapists is almost 8 000, and of healers around 20 000, compared with around 70 000 doctors in registered medical practice — the

reverse, in other words, of the Tanzanian situation.

Private, profit-making health care businesses range from individual practitioners to hospital chains and private insurance companies. The centre of private profit-making health care is often assumed to be the USA. The best-known American health insurance companies — Blue Cross and Blue Shield (the 'Blues') — are, however, incorporated as not-for-profit charitable organisations, while profit-making insurance carriers, of whom there are around 700, meet only 12–15 per cent of all health care expenditure. Only some 8 per cent of all American short-stay beds and 2 per cent of long-stay beds are in hospitals owned by profit-making organisations, but this still amounts to tens of thousands of beds, and some of the larger profit-making hospital chains are massive corporations by any standards: the largest, Humana Inc. of Louisville, Kentucky, had an annual turnover in 1984 of $2.61 billion, and an annual profit in the same year of $193 million.

In other countries, the proportion of all health care in the hands of profit-making organisations is often larger than in the USA. In Brazil, private hospitals, clinics, pharmacies, insurance companies and private-practice physicians account for almost two-thirds of total health expenditure. In Japan, 75 per cent of the country's 8 000 hospitals are owned by a combination of profit and non-profit making private owners, although most of the money to run them is paid from government or compulsory insurance sources.

In the UK, profit-making health care businesses are less

easy to identify: private insurers constitute around 5 per cent of total health care spending, but the main insurers in this area, like BUPA (the British United Provident Association), have a charitable status while being associated with profit-making subsidiaries. In India and Ghana profit-making activity tends to be confined to private medical practitioners working in the larger cities. Although China and the USSR do not officially favour private profit-making activity in health care or elsewhere, private practice still occurs. In other socialist countries, such as Czechoslovakia, the state permits a limited amount of private medical practice.

The role of *charitable and voluntary organisations* has been mentioned in relation to some Third World countries in the previous chapter. In Ghana, 34 of the country's 115 hospitals in 1971 were run by religious missions. In Brazil, charity hospitals number 1 200, ranging in size from 40 to 1 500 beds, and comprise the majority of the country's hospital provision. Traditionally they have been staffed by unpaid volunteers.

□ Earlier it was noted that around two-thirds of all recorded health care expenditure in Brazil is related to private profit-making activities. How can that figure be reconciled with the large number of hospitals that are not profit making?

■ The answer is simply that charitable and voluntary activity, because it is provided without formal payment, is not included in measures of health care expenditure.

Precisely because charitable and voluntary involvement in health care is often excluded from the standard accounts of health care spending, it is often underestimated. In fact, it continues to play a significant role in most countries. In the USSR, for example, the Red Cross and Red Crescent Societies contain 50 million voluntary members, or around one in five of the population. In addition, '. . . trade unions and women's and youth organisations are also involved. They help with radiography, and distribute health leaflets. Sanitary inspectors are also employed on a voluntary basis' (Hyde, 1974, p.200). These are routine uses of voluntary work, analogous to the dependence of many countries, such as the UK, on voluntary donations of blood. The USSR also makes use of occasional mass mobilisations in health care, such as the 'subbotnik' or voluntary Saturday work. One subbotnik in 1970, on the anniversary of Lenin's birthday, had the participation of 120 million people. These people either worked on health service projects — building, decorating, renovating hospitals, etc. — or contributed the wages from their own jobs. Voluntary mobilisations on a mass scale have also been used in China during particular health campaigns, in Cuba, and in Nicaragua. In the UK, one estimate of voluntary hospital activity suggested that the voluntary effort was equivalent to around 300 000 full-

time workers, spending around 50 per cent of their time on fund-raising and administration (CIPFA, 1984, p.33). And as we saw in earlier chapters, a small but important number of hospitals in Britain were run as voluntary hospitals until the inter-war years; in the USA some have survived to the present.

The category of *member-supported non-profit organisations* is separate only because the small number of organisations coming under this heading don't fit anywhere else! It refers to American Prepaid Group Practices (PPGPs), which began in the USA in the 1920s and are now better known as Health Maintenance Organisations (HMOs). Around 13 million Americans are in HMOs, the largest being the Californian Kaiser-Permanente Health Plan.

So what are they? HMOs are not strictly insurance organisations at all; indeed they are in a sense miniature national health services. Members pay in advance each month a flat-rate membership fee direct to the HMO, which in turn provides comprehensive health services to the members. The HMO is directly responsible for hospitals, doctors and so on, unlike insurance companies, which are intermediaries paying for these services without directly providing them. Because the HMO has a defined population of voluntarily enrolled members, and because members are restricted to care from the HMO's own facilities, it is often argued that the members and the HMOs both have incentives to keep the costs of services down, and that this contrasts with insurance systems, where the incentives are such as to push costs up.* One reason why this type of organisation might have an importance beyond its present size is that HMOs have been mooted repeatedly as a system of the future for the American health service as a whole.† However, the same was said of PPGPs in the 1920s.

Privately owned enterprises were noted in Chapter 7 as a typical way in which European health care was introduced to what were then colonies. A good example, described by Paul Basch, is the Volta Aluminium Company (VALCO) smelter in Tema, Ghana:

> Before 1958 Tema was a small fishing village. By 1962 it had 20 000 people; by 1972 it had 100 000 . . . The VALCO medical service began in 1964 with a compact ten-bed unit with laboratory, X-ray, and operating theatre, to serve some 3 000 construction workers. For the first three years of operation the service handled only work injuries; then it took over

---

*A fuller discussion of these issues is contained in *Caring for Health: Dilemmas and Prospects*, ibid. (U205 Book VIII).

†They are examined more closely in *Caring for Health: Dilemmas and Prospects*, ibid. (U205 Book VIII).

general health care of all employees. By 1969 service was extended to dependents of senior staff and the next year, with a work-force of 2 000, the company accepted responsibility for medical care of all dependents through a contract arrangement with a local clinic ... this sequence mirrors the historical developmental stages of many national programmes. (Basch, 1978, p.281)

The standard of care provided by many mine, plantation and other installation owners, however, particularly in Third World countries, was and remains very inadequate, while standards among local employers may often be even lower. In countries such as China and the USSR, industrial health care passed into state ownership along with the installations themselves. In Brazil and Nicaragua, occupation-based health services have developed in a different direction, towards occupation-based welfare funds or wider social insurance schemes, as discussed below. The provision of health services by private employers is still significant in many industrial countries, although again tends to be ignored. In the UK, around 5.5 per cent of private companies employ medical or nursing staff. Although the percentage is small, these companies together employ 52 per cent of the total labour force. In other words they are mainly large companies, though not necessarily particularly hazardous ones.

We come now to the two forms of health care organisation on which most attention tends to be focused: insurance-based health services and taxation based health services. Both involve insurance in the sense of protection by payment against risk of illness, but the methods of collection and distribution of funds are different.

Insurance against ill-health comes in many different forms. This diversity is explained largely by its historical origins in large numbers of separate sickness funds and societies organised around occupational groups, or residential areas, or religious bodies. In consequence, the development of sickness insurance has often been a story of different interest groups pulling in different directions: members of funds, the medical profession, and the government.

In Brazil, the numerous welfare funds, which had gradually grown to cover particular groups of workers, were amalgamated by government legislation in 1966 into a unified national administration, the Instituto Nacional de Presidencia Social (INPS). The consequence of this amalgamation was the extension of the medical services available to members of any one welfare fund to members of all funds, but because the medical services themselves — mainly physicians and hospitals — remained largely in private or charitable hands and were not similarly expanded, intense pressure on those services has developed.

Around one-third of the population, mainly in urban areas, is covered by the scheme.

In China, health care is based on a more comprehensive form of insurance. Factory workers, mainly in cities, are covered by health insurance paid by employers, a system also found in most East European countries. The Chinese scheme covers around 20 per cent of the population. The bulk of the Chinese population, in rural areas, are covered by local insurance schemes often operating at the level of communes. These local schemes work on the basis of a combination of annual fees for specific benefits, extra payments for some services, and local government subsidy. Although the problems are not comparable to those in Brazil, recent reports have suggested that the coverage of these schemes is wider than the services actually available, creating problems of access.

Voluntary insurance provides approximately 28 per cent of all health care expenditure in the USA, about one-half of this from profit-making insurers, as we saw earlier, and the other half from non-profit insurers.

☐ What central difficulty can you see in a health care system that is based solely on voluntary health insurance?

■ One central difficulty is that not everyone can afford the insurance premiums needed to obtain coverage and in particular that people who are old or in poor health (and therefore specially in need of health care) may be the least likely to be able to afford the higher payments they normally face.

It is this problem of restricted coverage in a voluntary health insurance system that has led to government intervention directed at groups who for one reason or another cannot get adequate insurance coverage against ill-health. In the United States, for example, the government finances medical programmes for Indians and armed forces veterans. The Veterans Administration by the late 1970s operated the largest centrally administered hospital system in the USA, providing medical care for 30 million veterans, or 14 per cent of the population. In addition, as part of the 'Great Society' programmes of the 1960s, the Federal government established a 'Medicaid' service for the poor, and a 'Medicare' service for the aged, both of these being groups which found difficulty in obtaining insurance coverage.

These programmes significantly extended the proportion of the population in the United States covered against ill-health. Although funded from taxation, these programmes are operated through the intermediary of the 'Blues'; in effect, the government pays for the insurance of people in the Medicare and Medicaid programmes. In 1984, Medicare provided hospital insurance protection to just under 30 million people (almost 14 per cent of the population). The medical programme is administered by individual states and varies considerably from one to another. California and New York, for example, have developed such broad medical programmes that they together spend 34 per cent of all Medicaid expenditure though they account for only 18 per cent of the total US population; Arizona, on the other hand, has no Medicaid programme. In total, 22.7 million people, or almost 11 per cent of the American population, were in receipt of Medicaid assistance in 1984; ten million of these were children under 21, another five million adults in poor families.

The government share of health care expenditure has been rising in America for a long time, from less than 15 per cent in 1930 to around 45 per cent in 1980. The years between 1965 and 1970 saw the most rapid increase, when the proportion of health care spending financed by the government rose from under 25 per cent to 37 per cent. It was during this period that the Medicare and Medicaid programmes were launched.

Despite these programmes, however, there are still major gaps in the 'coverage' of the American population: in 1978, of a total population of 220 million, 24 million (11 per cent) had no health insurance coverage at all from either the state or insurance companies, 19 million (9 per cent) had inadequate coverage, and 88 million (40 per cent) were not covered against what is referred to as 'catastrophic' illness: illnesses requiring very expensive treatments over a long/indefinite period (Maxwell, 1981, p.64).

One way of trying to overcome these coverage problems is to adopt some form of compulsory health insurance. Compulsory health insurance is now the dominant form of health care organisation in Europe, and voluntary insurance in these countries tends to be a way of obtaining extra benefits above those provided in the compulsory schemes.

The underlying trend in European countries operating compulsory health insurance schemes has been for the proportion of the population so covered to increase, as Table 8.1 shows.

Japan, which deliberately replaced Chinese medicine with German medicine in the nineteenth century, also imported the German system of health insurance. Since 1961 a compulsory social health insurance scheme has covered the entire population.

From such deep involvement by government in health care through insurance schemes, it seems in some ways but a small step to move to a comprehensive system of health care covering the entire population and provided directly by government. In fact, such *national taxation-based health services* exist in only a small number of countries, and, as Chapter 5 showed with the example of the British National Health Service, the circumstances under which

Table 8.1 The increased coverage of health insurance in eight European countries (%)

Country	Coverage in	
	1966	1975
Belgium	75	85
Denmark	90	100
West Germany	86	90
Ireland	39	85
France	94	98
Italy	85	94
Luxembourg	99	99
Netherlands	70	70

(Source: derived from Abel-Smith and Maynard, 1978)

they have been established have tended to be exceptional. In the USSR the central organisational form of health care after the 1917 revolution was social health insurance, a system which lasted for about twenty years. In the 1930s a widening range of treatments was being provided by the state irrespective of any insurance qualifications, and by the post-war period almost all health care was financed directly from state budgets. If a date is to be sought, therefore, for the first national health service, the best candidate is 1937 when social health insurance was abolished in the USSR.

The formation of the NHS in Britain in 1948 has already been discussed. The example of the NHS was influential in a number of British ex-colonies. In India, the Report of the Health Survey and Development Committee (the Bhore Report) proposed in 1946 that:

(1) No one should fail to secure adequate medical care because of inability to pay for it; (2) The health programme must from the very beginning lay emphasis on preventative work; (3) Health services should be placed as close to the people as possible; (4) The doctor of the future should be a social physician; (5) Medical services should be free to all without distinction and the contribution from those who can afford to pay should be through general and local taxation ... (Ramalingaswarmi, 1973, p.195)

This statement of intent still guides health policy-making in India, but has never been fulfilled for, among other reasons, lack of money to provide such a service. The same obstacle has been encountered in Ghana, where, as a former director of Ghanaian medical services wrote, there was a belief at independence in 1957 '... that central government alone would finance all health services for the people. This has led to a state of affairs where for about two US dollars per head per year [1973] the government has been expected to provide free general service to everybody' (Sai, 1973, p.137). As in Chile, where a national health service covering hospital services was established in 1952, the Ghanaian system, whatever its shortcomings, was finally ended as a result of a military coup, in itself a reaction against wider social and economic policies. In Cuba, by contrast, it was the political revolution of 1958 that led to the creation of a national health service run by central, provincial, regional and local government, as in the USSR.

Other countries operating some form of national health service include New Zealand and, since 1979, Italy. There is no standard pattern: in Sweden the costs of many health care items are met through social insurance, but hospitals have been publicly owned since the 1920s. And, whereas in the UK the tax revenue that funds the NHS is raised on a purely national basis, in Sweden over 95 per cent of the taxation revenue needed to run the health services is raised locally.

It is evident, then, that the range of organisational forms that exist to provide formal health care is wide, and that different types of provision can simultaneously exist. Can we therefore make comparisons between such different systems? In practice, the most common response to this diversity has been to focus attention on specific topics in specific countries. In western industrialised countries, a particular focus of attention has been on the cost of formal health care.

The cost of formal health care

Formal health services now consume somewhere between 5 per cent and 10 per cent of the total national wealth of the richest industrialised countries. Moreover, this share has been growing steadily: in the 1950s, the average share taken by formal health care in these same countries was around 4 per cent.

As formal health care expenditure has grown, so too has concern by governments, and 'cost-containment' policies have become widespread, although with varying degrees of success. Associated with these policies, doubts have increasingly been voiced about the *value* obtained from health care expenditure.

In a sense, this concern over the value of formal health care expenditure is a continuation of a long-standing debate on the effect of formal health care on health. Seen in this way, the cost of health care is just one side of an equation which includes on the other side, the results, benefits, output or contribution of health care.

We will come to the other side of this equation shortly, but a starting point would be to establish how many resources are devoted to formal health care in different countries. A way of attempting to measure this is to try to express the total amount spent on formal health care as a sum per head of population, converted into a standard currency so that different countries can be compared. Figure 8.2 shows the results of such an exercise conducted for ten countries in 1977.

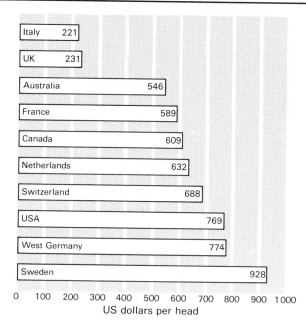

Figure 8.2 Health care expenditure in ten countries, 1977 (US dollars per head)
(Source: Maxwell, 1981, Fig. 3.2, p.35)

The ten countries shown in Figure 8.2 are in many ways very similar: industrialised, western European or of European origin, and wealthy in relation to most of the world. Even within this group, however, there are wide differences in the amount spent each year on formal health care per person: over four times as much in Sweden as in Italy, for example.

Many different reasons could be given for these differences. In the first place, it is probable that like is not being compared with like. There are differences in what counts as formal health care in different countries. For example, running a formal health care system involves the training and education of many personnel. In Canada, nursing education is provided in community colleges and is excluded from health spending, as it is in Sweden and the USA. In the other countries in Figure 8.2, however, education of nurses and other staff is largely included. The population covered in each country also varies: in West Germany the reported expenditure figure excludes health services for the armed forces, in the other countries they are included.

☐ In what other areas would you particularly expect there to be international differences in what is referred to as formal health care?
■ One of the vaguest boundaries is between formal health care and the social welfare services.

A wide range of social welfare services are included as

formal health care in some countries but excluded in others. Among these are those for drug addicts, for the physically and mentally handicapped, residential and private nursing homes for the elderly, and community services for alcoholics. The list of these discrepancies could be extended: in the French figures, personal travel costs to and from hospital and the costs of clinic or doctor are included; in Switzerland, the figures don't even include ambulances. However, although these differences do cast light on the way in which the boundaries of formal health care vary, they have been shown to explain only a small proportion of the variation in spending shown in Figure 8.2.

Another difficulty involved in making international comparisons like those in Figure 8.2 arises from the need to convert expenditures measured in national currencies into one standard form.

    ☐ Why might this be a problem?
    ■ Exchange rates between currencies can fluctuate sharply over short periods, and this can distort comparisons between countries.

In Figure 8.2 the expenditure in each country was converted into dollars using the average exchange rate in 1977. But between 1976 and 1978 the dollar exchange rate rose in Switzerland by 62 per cent, rose in the Netherlands by 36 per cent, rose in West Germany by 44 per cent, and fell in Canada by 14 per cent and in Italy by 17 per cent. Clearly, if the expenditure figures shown in the figure had been calculated in 1976 or 1978 using different exchange rates, the pattern would have changed by substantially more than any actual change in the amount of formal health care provided.

One way of avoiding problems with exchange rates is to look instead at the proportion of national wealth devoted to formal health care in different countries. This is normally done by expressing health expenditure as a percentage of a country's total national wealth, as measured by its Gross National Product (GNP).

Figure 8.3 shows formal health care expenditure as a proportion of GNP for the same ten countries listed in Figure 8.2. (The figures are for 1977, which at the time of writing was the most recent year for which reasonably reliable figures had been calculated.)

    ☐ Comparing Figures 8.2 and 8.3, what similarities and differences strike you?
    ■ The ranking of the ten countries remains broadly similar, but the magnitude of difference between countries is less.

Since 1977, estimates suggest that these figures have tended to rise, and that the UK in 1984 was spending about 6 per cent of its GNP on formal health care, rising to between 10 and 12.5 per cent of GNP in the USA and West Germany.

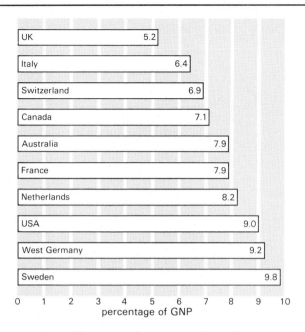

Figure 8.3 Health care expenditure as a proportion of GNP in ten countries, 1977
(Source: Maxwell, 1981, Fig. 3.5, p.38)

Even in this small group of countries, therefore, the proportion of total national wealth devoted to formal health care can vary by upwards of a factor of two.

Among all the countries shown in Figure 8.3 there has been a general trend since the 1960s towards formal health care taking a larger and larger slice of national wealth, and it was suggested earlier in the chapter that this rise was one reason why attention has increasingly focused on international comparisons of costs.

One obvious reason for variations between countries in the absolute amount spent on formal health care is that countries vary in their total wealth, and so in the USA more is spent on formal health care than in the UK, just as more is spent on clothes or housing or motors or food, because the USA is a country where the average level of personal wealth is significantly higher than in the UK. Up to a point this is certainly true, but what is interesting is not that wealthier countries spend more, but that wealthier countries systematically devote a larger and larger *proportion* of their wealth to formal health care. If the USA, Sweden or West Germany were all devoting the same proportion of their GNP to formal health care as the UK, health care spending per person would be a lot higher in these countries than in the UK because their GNP is in fact higher than the UK's. But the *proportion* of GNP these three countries devote to formal health care is roughly twice that of the UK making their spending much more than twice as much per person, as Figure 8.2 shows.

Table 8.2 Health care resources in nine countries (1981 or nearest date for which data are available)

Country	GNP per capita (US $) 1982	Public expenditure on health as a % of GNP	Health expenditure per capita (US $)
Nepal	170	0.5	1
India	260	0.2	1
China	310	—	—
Ghana	360	0.7	3
Nicaragua	920	4.4	41
Brazil	2 240	1.4	32
UK	9 660	5.6	541
Japan	10 080	—	—
USA	13 160	8.3	1 092

(Source: derived from World Bank, 1984, Tables 1, 24 and 26, pp.218–9, 264–5, 268–9)

It seems clear, then, that one important reason why different countries spend varying amounts on formal health care is that they vary in their level of total wealth. Indeed, it has been suggested that total wealth is far and away the best predictor of formal health care spending. An American researcher, Joseph Newhouse, found that in his sample of thirteen industrialised countries over 90 per cent of the variation in formal health care spending per person could be statistically 'explained' by variations in per capita wealth (Newhouse, 1977). Findings such as this do convey an important message: that there seems to be no ceiling or limit to how much can be spent on formal health care and the richer a country becomes the more it will tend to spend. Conversely, it could be predicted from these findings that the poorer a country is, the less it will spend on health. How true is this? Table 8.2 shows the per capita national income of a sample of countries, alongside the proportion of total GNP spent by the government on formal health care and what this government-funded health care represents in US dollars per capita.

□ In light of the previous discussion of different forms of health care organisation and provision, what strikes you about the health care included in this table?
■ It only covers *government* expenditure on health care, omitting many other categories: charitable, private, etc.

Despite these limitations, it seems clear from the table that in poorer countries formal health care spending per person is a tiny fraction of what is spent in countries such as the UK or USA. With only a few dollars per person to spend each year on formal health care, and with far greater health problems, the obstacles faced by many countries are obvious.

So far, we have been comparing *average* levels of formal health care spending per person in different countries, but there are also substantial variations in the way this is distributed *within* countries.

An example of this is given in Table 8.3, which compares the way that hospital expenditure is spread among regions of France, the Netherlands and England.

□ How would you summarise this comparison?
■ The figures show that in England the 'best endowed' region of the country received 13 per cent more hospital resources than it might expect if these resources were equally shared across all regions, and the 'worst endowed' region received 9 per cent less. In the Netherlands the best endowed and worst endowed regions were both further away from the 'equal share' than in England, and in France the differences were very wide indeed — the best endowed region receiving almost one-third more than a fair share, and the worst receiving 57 per cent less than might be expected.

It was shown earlier that both the Netherlands and France spend more on health than the UK; as the table shows, they also seem to distribute it more unequally than in England. Regional differences in expenditure are only one form of inequality in health care *within* nations, but they do illustrate the shortcomings of relying on very simple measures when making international comparisons.

Health care 'inputs'

Given the existence of such large international variations in the total amount and the pattern of formal health care expenditure, it is to be expected that significant differences will also exist between countries in the numbers of doctors, nurses, hospitals and beds — that is, the 'inputs' used to produce formal health care. In fact, there is no simple relationship between expenditure and these 'inputs', and an

Table 8.3 Regional inequalities in hospital expenditure in England, France and the Netherlands.

| Country | Distance away from 'fair share' of expenditure as percentage of actual expenditure in | |
	best endowed region	worst endowed region
England (1979–80)	+ 13	− 9
Netherlands (1976)	+ 14	− 23
France (1977)	+ 31	− 57

(Source: Maynard and Ludbrook, 1981, Table 4, p.62)

even more complicated relationship between the 'inputs' which are provided and the amount of formal health care 'activity' taking place. Table 8.4, for example, shows the population per physician and per nurse in thirteen countries in 1980.

Japan, with a population per physician of 780, is one of the least doctored of industrialised countries, followed by the UK. By comparison Italy has almost twice as many doctors as the UK, relative to population, and the USSR, where one in every 280 citizens is a doctor, has more than any other country in the world. At the other extreme are countries like Ghana and Nepal, where for each physician there are thousands or tens of thousands of people.

☐ The right-hand column of the table shows the population per nurse in the same thirteen countries. Is there an obvious association between this and the provision of doctors?

■ There is a general tendency for there to be more nurses where there are more doctors, but there are several important exceptions. Italy, for example, has a

high number of doctors but a very low number of nurses: in fact, approximately one nurse per doctor. And in China there is also approximately one nurse per doctor, but in Ghana ten times as many nurses as doctors and in India more doctors than nurses.

Even less comparative research has been done on nurses than doctors, and so the reasons for these variations — and the implications — are still very imperfectly understood.

There are many views on the appropriate balance of different types of health workers. But, as with average levels of expenditure, it can be misleading to focus on average numbers of doctors or nurses within a country. In particular, enormous differences can exist between rural and urban areas: in the 1960s, Addis Ababa, capital of Ethiopia, had 2.5 per cent of the country's population, but 50 per cent of all its doctors; Bangkok, one doctor per 940 people compared with one per 200 000 in rural areas of Thailand; Bombay, Calcutta and New Delhi one doctor per 500 people, but in rural areas one per 30 000–45 000. Not surprisingly, in many countries large portions of the population are effectively not provided with any formal health care: in Ghana, for example, detailed investigation '... indicated that a third to a half of the population of the districts investigated lived outside the effective reach of the health units providing basic health care and that the services provided were generally of low quality' (Mills, 1983, p.1973).

Doctors and nurses are only one part of formal health care, and systematic information on other aspects of formal health services is less easy to find for a wide range of countries. Figure 8.4 (overleaf) displays data on two other aspects of formal health care: the number of hospital beds available and the average length of stay of people admitted to general hospitals.

Table 8.4 Number of people per physician and per nurse in thirteen countries (1980)

| Country | Population per | |
	Registered physician	Nurse
USSR	270	100
Italy	340	330
USA	520	140
UK	650	140
Cuba	710	360
Japan	780	240
Brazil (1977)	1 700	822
Nicaragua	1 800	550
China	1 810	1 790
India	3 690	5 460
Ghana	7 630	780
Nepal	30 060	33 420

(Source: World Bank, 1984, Table 24, pp.264–5)

☐ How might you expect these two measures to be related?

■ Short lengths of stay may make it possible to treat the same number of patients with fewer beds, and vice versa.

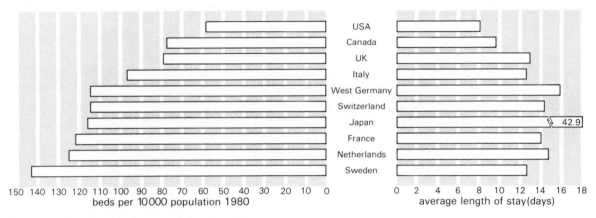

Figure 8.4 Beds and length of stay in ten countries, 1980

The figure does indeed show that these two measures appear to be positively related: thus the USA makes do with half the beds per 10 000 population than West Germany, where the length of stay is twice as long. It has been calculated that by bringing its lengths of stay into line with those prevailing in the USA, the French hospital system could dispense with 45 per cent of its total bed capacity (OECD, 1977, p.71).

Why these differences exist, however, is again complex and not well understood. To some extent the number of hospital beds will be influenced by the availability of other kinds of service that might keep people out of hospital. Indeed, it has been estimated that up to 60 per cent of old people in European mental hospitals could be cared for outside hospital, if such services existed (OECD, 1977, p.70). But the relation between hospital provision and lay care has not received serious international attention. Similarly, the length of stay might be expected to be influenced by the quality and coverage of other forms of care: it would be easier, for example, to discharge a patient more rapidly from hospital if home nursing and home help services were available. However, such services are better developed in the UK, with longer lengths of stay, than in the USA, which has very short lengths of stay.

The USA is at present moving towards a policy of laying down standard lengths of stay.

☐ Who would you consider to be most likely to wish to do this?

■ The main organisations pushing for this are the federal agencies such as Medicare which pay hospitals for a substantial proportion of their patients.

The Medicare programme has increasingly tried to control its expenditure by fixing rates of reimbursement for hospital stays for particular diagnoses, irrespective of the actual length of stay. In Eastern Europe, too, lengths of stay are often administratively prescribed for major causes of admission, so that a patient admitted to hospital in the USSR for the removal of an appendix might automatically be kept in for, say, twelve days. Where these norms have not been imposed, however, it is known that lengths of stay vary considerably within countries, and indeed between consultants in the same hospitals. It has been suggested that the way in which hospitals are financed is one factor influencing lengths of stay: many western European hospitals are refunded their running costs by insurance companies on the basis of a set rate per patient day. This 'per diem' financing system is particularly common in West Germany and France, where average lengths of stay are comparatively long, but a similar system is also familiar in parts of the American hospital system where stays are short: so clearly other factors must also be taken into account.

There is very little evidence about either the clinical effectiveness or the cost implications of different lengths of stay; the fact that so much variation does exist strongly underlines the absence of any 'normal' or 'natural' treatment pattern. Indeed, it has been suggested that the amount of treatment provided will be strongly influenced by the means available: that supply creates its own demand. For example, it has been pointed out that a 'shortage' of doctors will not necessarily be removed by increasing the numbers of doctors. Thus in Canada it was found that a steady increase in the supply of doctors seemed to do nothing towards reducing the workload per doctor: each 5 per cent increase in the number of doctors increased total workload by over 4 per cent. Similarly, Figure 8.5 shows an increase of over 40 per cent in ear, nose and throat surgeons in England and Wales between 1965 and 1981, but a fall of less than 20 per cent in waiting lists.

What might explain this? In most instances where goods or services are being exchanged, the roles of the person

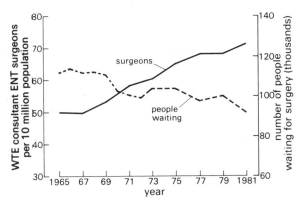

Figure 8.5 Changes in numbers of ENT surgeons and size of waiting lists, England and Wales, 1965–1981.

demanding and the person *supplying* are taken by two people assumed to be equally well informed. The patient 'demanding' formal health care, however, is frequently in a bad position to know what to demand.

☐ Why might this be so?
■ First, the patient may be unconscious or in need of emergency treatment. Second, the patient will frequently be at a disadvantage over information: about what is wrong, what sort of treatments are available and their likely consequences, or even whether treatment is good or bad.

In short, there is an *asymmetry* in the information available to doctor and patient, which results in the doctor making decisions about what to supply to the patient. The doctor can be said to be inducing a demand for her or his own services. This phenomenon, for which the Canadian economist, R.G. Evans, has found widespread evidence, has come to be called '*supplier-induced demand*' (Evans, 1974), and carries important implications for formal health care provision, for if it is widely occurring, the idea of a 'shortage' of formal health care takes on new meaning: the more formal health care is supplied the more will be demanded.

☐ What circumstances can you think of in which doctors might have particular incentives to create supplier-induced demand?
■ If they are paid according to the number of services that they provide, then they will have a financial incentive to induce as much demand for their services as possible.

The payment of doctors according to the services they perform is called a '*fee-for-service*' payment system, and is essentially a form of piece-rate. Fee-for-service payment is

common in many countries, although the details vary considerably and the impact of the system may therefore take different forms. In Japan, for example, the payment system is such that doctors make profits from the volume of pharmaceuticals supplied. This has led to accusations that excessive prescribing and injecting occurs. In West Germany, doctors can claim for X-rays and anaesthetics, and the result has been not only accusations of high rates of X-ray use, but also, because doctors monopolise such work, very low numbers of radiologists and anaesthetists.

The controversy over supplier-induced demand and the effects of fee-for-service payment systems has waxed particularly strongly over rates of surgery in different countries. Figure 8.6 shows operation rates covering seven procedures in England and Wales, the USA and the Saskatchewan province of Canada.

The variations shown in Figure 8.6 do not seem to be related to differential disease incidence, yet the hysterectomy rate is three times higher in Saskatchewan than in the UK, and the rate of hernia repair in the USA is almost double the rate in the UK. Similar examples can be found in other countries: thus the West German appendicectomy rate is approximately three times the rate in the UK or the USA.

The reasons for surgical intervention are many and complex.* Nevertheless, it is fairly clear that the existence of a fee-for-service payment system, as in West Germany or the USA, has some influence over the rates of surgical intervention compared with rates in the UK where surgeons are paid by a salary that is independent of the volume of work done. Moreover, it seems that by increasing the supply of formal health care one also increases the demand, so that in the USA, the number of surgeons per capita and the number of surgical operations are both double the comparable figures in the UK. Finally, it is plausible to suggest that such variations are connected to different levels of income. In high-income countries such as the USA, operations may be purchased when they offer some measure of reassurance to the patient, who may have no symptoms. The spectre of 'preventive mastectomy' is alarming, but equally, in a society familiar with the horrors of cancer, it would be an economically 'rational' choice for someone terrified of the disease, having a great need for reassurance, and having a high enough income to pay for it.

*Hysterectomy is discussed in much more detail in *Medical Knowledge: Doubt and Certainty*, *ibid.* Appendicectomy is similarly discussed in *Experiencing and Explaining Disease*, *ibid.* (U205 Books II and VI).

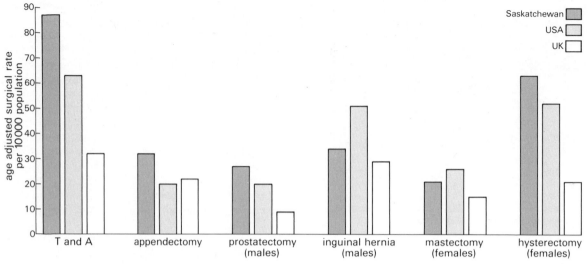

Figure 8.6 Operation rates in three countries, 1969–1971

(Source: Bunker, *et al.*, 1977, Table 7.8, p.100)

Health care and health

The extent to which the amount of formal health care provided seems to be influenced by such things as income, wealth, and insurance or payment systems, gives rise to perhaps the most important question of all: what effect does formal health care actually have on health? Table 8.5 shows ten industrialised countries ranked to the left according to the percentage of GNP they spend on formal health care, and to the right by their rating on a standardised mortality index (based on a comparison of seventeen age and sex-specific death rates in each country against the mean rates for all ten countries). In effect, the table is an attempt to compare the resources going into formal health care — the 'inputs' — with what might be seen as one of the consequences or 'outputs' of health care — the level of health.

☐ What strikes you about the positions each country holds in these two rankings?

■ There seems to be very little connection between them. Countries such as West Germany and the USA are top spenders on formal health care but are bottom in the mortality index rating. By contrast, Switzerland and the UK come out well when ranked by the mortality index, but are at the bottom of the league in terms of the proportion of their GNP spent on formal health care.

This same apparent lack of connection between formal health care and mortality is shown in Figure 8.7. In this figure, fifteen countries have been arranged in ascending order from left to right according to the percentage increase in the share of GNP they devoted to formal health care

Table 8.5 Levels of formal health care spending and mortality in ten countries

| Country | Rank, according to | |
	Percentage of GNP spent on formal health care	Standardised mortality index
Sweden	1	1
West Germany	2	10
USA	3	9
Netherlands	4	2
France	5	7
Australia	6	5
Canada	7	6
Switzerland	8	3
Italy	9	8
UK	10	4

(Source: derived from Figure 8.5, and Maxwell, 1981, Tables 3–4, p.52)

between 1962 and 1975, ranging from a 12 per cent increase in Belgium to a 40 per cent increase in the Netherlands. The dotted line in the figure shows the percentage decline in the infant mortality rate in each country over approximately the same period.

☐ If increasing formal health care resources did have a direct effect on mortality, what pattern might you expect these two lines in Figure 8.7 to follow?

■ The two lines might be expected to move upwards together; that is, bigger increases in formal health care

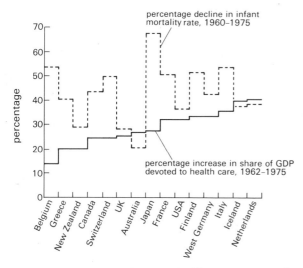

Figure 8.7 A comparison of changing health care resources and changing health in fifteen countries

(Source: OECD, 1979, Tables 11 and 17, pp.28 and 49)

resources should be accompanied by bigger reductions in infant mortality rates.

☐ Can you see any such obvious relationship between the two lines?

■ There doesn't appear to be one. The dotted line fluctuates sharply and shows no trend.

In Figure 8.7 there is no obvious association between formal health care and mortality. However, in a study of eighteen industrialised countries, the epidemiologist, Archie Cochrane, and two colleagues did find an association; but they found not only that none of their measures of health care provision was inversely related to mortality, but that a strong *positive* relationship existed between the prevalence of doctors in a country and mortality rates! The study did not claim that this was a causal relationship, but to have the prevalence of doctors placed alongside cigarette and alcohol consumption as the main factors positively associated with mortality was embarrassment enough (Cochrane, St Leger and Moore, 1978).

What does this apparent lack of correspondence between health care and mortality mean? There are many difficulties involved in trying to assess the relationship between health care and health. First, the measurement of health care resources produces many problems, as discussed earlier in this chapter. Second, just because a country spends a lot on health care and does not have comparably low mortality rates, it does not follow that the

health care was ineffectual: mortality rates might have been even higher without large amounts of health care. And third, we are only assessing the effect of health care in terms of mortality, which might be quite unrealistic. The problem is that it is so much more difficult to measure morbidity, or reductions in anxiety, or comfort, reassurance and 'tender loving care'.

Despite such measurement problems, it is evident that it is necessary to consider much more than mortality rates when assessing the effect of formal health care. A significant number of activities are in no way intended to reduce mortality — hip replacement, for example, is an area of formal health care provision that is intended primarily to improve the *quality* of life.

In addition, there is now virtually no limit to the amount of intensive care that can be provided to a patient in the last stages of life, with a negligible effect on survival chances: failing breathing can be countered by mechanical respirators, failing kidneys with renal dialysis machines. Modern anaesthetics and surgical techniques make it possible to operate on the very old, when gains in life expectancy may be extremely small. Particular ethical and legal issues arise in relation to how much medical care should be given to the very old, or in the more dramatic language of much debate, when to 'switch the machines off', for such care may make dying more bearable.

But even if it is assumed that 'switching off the machine' is a fairly widespread practice in hospitals in many countries, fabulous sums of money may still be involved; it emerged during a debate in the American House of Representatives Ways and Means Committee, for example, that Medicare in 1983 spent 15 billion dollars on providing care for old people in their last six months of life. This seems to be part of a more general tendency, to adopt technologically sophisticated and highly expensive forms of medical care whose effectiveness is unproven or known to be small. For example, the survival chances of most people who have suffered a heart attack are not significantly affected by attention in an intensive care unit. One description of heroic endeavour on behalf of the patient whose illness seems wellnigh hopeless is to be found in *The Family Reunion* by T.S. Eliot, where a plea is entered that something be done,

Not for the good that it will do,
But that nothing may be left undone
On the margin of the impossible.

The overall volume of spending on formal health care, on this account, may have little direct connection with health, in part because so much of it, in some countries at least, is on this 'margin of the impossible'.

Objectives for Chapter 8

When you have finished studying this chapter, you should be able to:

8.1 Describe the main ways in which the finance of formal health care may be organised.

8.2 Discuss trends in the resources committed to formal health care between different countries, and the difficulties involved in making comparisons.

8.3 Describe some of the principal measures of formal health care 'inputs' and activities, and some reasons why they might vary between countries.

8.4 Summarise the debate over the relationship between formal health care and health in industrialised countries, and the evidence furnished by recent studies.

Questions for Chapter 8

1 (*Objective 8.1*) Formal health care systems based on insurance seem often to be characterised by the large number of organisations involved. What explanations can you offer for this?

2 (*Objective 8.2*) 'Spending on formal health care increases in direct line with national wealth.' Is this statement true?

3 (*Objective 8.3*) Under what circumstances might a 'shortage' of doctors not be overcome by increasing the number of doctors at work?

4 (*Objective 8.4*) Why might you expect the connection between mortality rates and the amount of formal health care provided to be weak?

9

Formal health care: models and practice

During this chapter you will be referred to the Course Reader for the articles 'Traditional Indian medicine in practice in an Indian metropolitan city' written by A. Ramesh and B. Hyma, and 'The village health worker: lackey or liberator?' written by David Werner (Part 4, Section 4.3 and Part 3, Section 3.10).

In the previous chapter we saw that it was possible to impose a broad framework of classification on the many different ways of financing formal health care. By comparing the amount of resources going into formal health care in different countries, we were able to conclude that the quantity of formal health care that any country supports seems to be determined primarily by that country's overall level of national wealth. The final lesson to emerge from the chapter was that the quantity of formal health care in a country does not seem to be related to levels of health, at least as measured by mortality rates or life expectancy.

In this chapter, we shall continue the task of classification and analysis, focusing now on the organisation of services within formal health care, and on the relation between these services and the problems of ill-health that they face. What analytical devices can we make use of to examine these aspects of formal health care, and what can we learn from them?

Levels of health care

As you have seen, one feature of the organisation of health care in industrialised countries such as Britain has been the increasing degree of *specialisation*, both between and within occupational groups, hospitals and other institutions.

The least specialised part of the NHS, in the sense that it caters for people of all ages and with any condition, is *primary care*. This is the point at which people make first contact with the health service. In the UK the mainstay of primary care is general practice. However, it also includes other basic services for particular groups such as school health, occupational health, and community clinics for family planning and child health. In addition, much of the work of hospital accident and emergency departments can be considered as part of primary care. Not only are primary care services essentially *generalist* in nature, but their other key feature is that people have access to them without having to be referred by a doctor, a process termed *self-referral*.

This is not true of other parts of the NHS in Britain. If a primary care doctor considers that the opinion of a more specialised doctor is required, a patient will be referred to another part of the system, called *secondary care*. In the NHS, secondary care is largely organised in District General Hospitals (DGHs), each one serving a population of about 250 000 people. Secondary care encompasses all the basic specialities such as medicine, surgery, obstetrics, gynaecology, paediatrics, orthopaedics and ear, nose and throat surgery.

If a patient requires even more specialised care, she or he may be referred to yet another part of the NHS, that can be termed *tertiary care*. This includes such services as plastic surgery, cardiac surgery, renal dialysis or spinal injuries.* As people seldom require such services, tertiary care is organised on a regional basis, serving populations of several million.

It can be seen, therefore, that one way of coming to grips with the great variety of services offered by the NHS is to think in terms of *level of specialisation*: from the primary care level through the secondary care level to the tertiary care level. And with this very simple model, we can then ask questions about *access* and *distribution*; for example, what arrangements exist for people to obtain services at different levels, who else is involved in making decisions about access, or how formal health care resources are distributed between these three levels.

Moreover, this three-level model need not correspond to any actual administrative divisions in the country's formal health services. It is simply a device that enables us to compare the various services that exist in different countries by seeing how they fit into the model.

Let's illustrate this by considering briefly three other countries: the USSR, USA and Japan. Unlike the UK, primary care is relatively undeveloped in these three countries. Instead of referring themselves to a generalist family doctor, people have to seek directly the help of a specialist. In the USSR, such specialists work in groups in polyclinics. Polyclinics, which were first established in the 1880s, are sometimes (though not always) on the same site as a hospital. In some ways the Soviet model is similar to that in the USA where people refer themselves to specialists whose offices, for consultations, are often grouped together

in medical buildings that are not dissimilar to polyclinics.

Of course, similarities in organisation need not mean that services are provided in the same way; other things such as methods of payment also affect access. For example, whereas in the USSR everyone has access to specialists at the polyclinics, in the USA not everyone can afford to consult a specialist in the way described. For such people, an alternative service is available in the out-patient departments of the large city hospitals which act as 'safety nets' to catch those people who would otherwise be unable to get medical assistance.

☐ Can you recall a similar arrangement existing in Britain at anytime?
■ In the eighteenth and nineteenth centuries, when out-patient departments for the poor expanded in some of the voluntary hospitals.

The need for some form of 'safety net' is not entirely a thing of the past in Britain. Accident and emergency departments currently provide a similar service in some inner city areas in which general practice is inadequate.

As with the USSR and USA, Japan also lacks a system of generalist family doctors so that people either have to consult private specialists or refer themselves to the out-patient department of a hospital.

All three countries have recently tried to develop a form of primary care similar to that in the UK. In the USSR attempts to establish 'sector doctors' with a general responsibility for the whole population resident in one sector, such as a single housing estate, have largely been

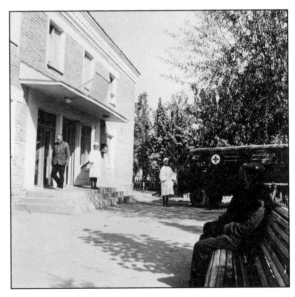

Figure 9.1 The polyclinic of the number 17 State Farm in the Hungry Steppe of Tajik Soviet Socialist Republic.

*You should be aware that 'tertiary care' is sometimes used in a different way to mean the long-term hospital care provided for chronically sick or infirm people. This is not the meaning used in this book.

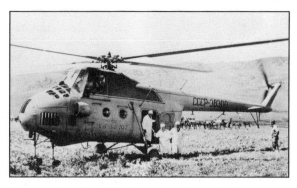

Figure 9.2 One-third of the Russian population live in non-urban areas, where health services are often poorer. In this photo, medical personnel from the Susamyrsky Divisional Hospital in Kingistan Republic are visiting cattle men in the mountain pastures of Symaryr, using a helicopter of the Health Aviation Service.

unsuccessful. This seems to have been because the posts lacked authority: patients can and do continue to consult specialists at the polyclinic. Although Soviet health planners recognise the value of a single generalist doctor with a continuing responsibility for people, doctors continue to be trained as specialists. Changes in the pattern of care therefore are unlikely to come about unless other changes occur in medical education, training and recruitment.

In the USA and Japan progress in developing generalists has also been limited, and it seems unlikely that there will be any dramatic change in the future. What are the obstacles in these countries? An essential aspect of both countries' formal health care systems is *private provision*, where the patient decides on which doctor to consult. In a generalist system, the family doctor makes the decision as to whether a specialist opinion is necessary, and if so, which speciality and which doctor to consult. But in a private system based on consumer choice, generalist doctors would be an anachronism.

Differences also exist in the pattern of secondary and tertiary care. Referral from polyclinic to hospital in USSR is reminiscent of the NHS. The hospitals are organised on a similar basis, ranging from small town and urban district institutions to large ones serving whole regions and republics. In addition to general hospitals providing a similar range of specialities as in a DGH in the UK, there are specialised hospitals for tertiary care. Although the organisation of secondary and tertiary care in the USSR and UK is similar, the extent to which each is used differs. In the USSR there is much greater emphasis on hospital care — patients who would be treated at home or as out-patients in the UK are often placed in hospital in the USSR.

  ☐ Can you think of any *geographical* explanations for this?

  ■ The UK is a much smaller and more urbanised country than the USSR, and people can more easily travel to and from a hospital in a day.

Whereas in the UK and USSR doctors work predominantly either in primary or in secondary care, in the USA the same doctor will often be both the patient's point of first contact with the health service *and* the provider of specialist, secondary care. A further difference is that if another doctor's skills are required, the patient is not actually *referred* to a specific doctor, but simply *advised* as to which specialist to consult: the choice of specialist rests with the patient.

  ☐ As you have seen in Chapter 8, there are some exceptions to this arrangement in the USA. What are they?
  ■ Health Maintenance Organisations (HMOs).

As members can only be seen by HMO doctors, a referral, rather than an advisory, system operates.

With the exception of the HMOs, hospitals in the USA compete with one another commercially. One consequence of this is that despite repeated attempts, there is little regional planning of hospital services. Far from dispersing, in many cities hospitals have tended to congregate in one area. The same is true in Japan where the idea of avoiding duplication of services by organising hospitals on a regional basis had been rejected up to the 1970s, and by the mid-1980s had still not been realised.

So far, we have seen how the primary–secondary–tertiary model can be applied to industrialised countries. How well does it fit countries in the Third World? In the Course Reader an article by Ramesh and Hyma discusses aspects of medical practice in the southern Indian city of Madras. Read this article now,* and then consider the following questions.

  ☐ What proportions of health care are estimated to be provided by indigenous practitioners, western medicine, and lay care?
  ■ About 40 per cent by indigenous practitioners, 20 per cent by western medicine, and 40 per cent by lay care.
  ☐ How specialised were the indigenous practitioners?
  ■ There appeared to be little formal specialisation, and most practitioners treated a wide range of disorders.
  ☐ How did patients obtain access to these practitioners?
  ■ They self-referred, and paid a fee for each visit.

*Ramesh, A. and Hyma, B., 'Traditional Indian Medicine in Practice in an Indian Metropolitan City', in Black, N., *et al.* (eds), *ibid.*

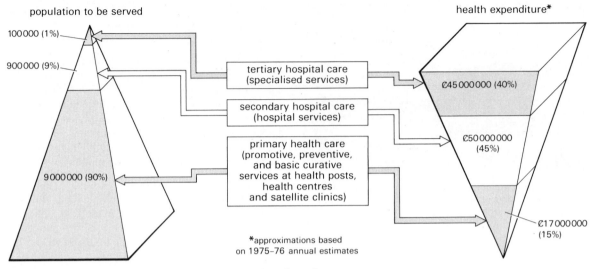

population to be served

100 000 (1%)

900 000 (9%)

9 000 000 (90%)

health expenditure*

tertiary hospital care
(specialised services)

secondary hospital care
(hospital services)

primary health care
(promotive, preventive,
and basic curative
services at health posts,
health centres
and satellite clinics)

₵45 000 000 (40%)

₵50 000 000
(45%)

₵17 000 000
(15%)

*approximations based
on 1975–76 annual estimates

Figure 9.3 The mismatch between health care resources and needs in Ghana, 1978.

□   How might these practitioners fit into the primary–secondary–tertiary model?

■   They seem to have many of the characteristics of a primary care system.

Earlier in the book, we saw that in pre-industrial Europe most people also relied on a wide range of traditional or indigenous practitioners, whose skills and mode of practice were probably similar in many respects to those studied by Ramesh and Hyma. We also saw that, although hospitals and infirmaries existed in pre-industrial Europe, it was during the rapid industrial expansion of the nineteenth century that hospital building occurred on an unprecedented scale — the secondary and tertiary levels of health care were a product of industrialisation.

So in many Third World countries we might predict that, although there might be a fairly large primary care sector provided by indigenous practitioners, the secondary and tertiary levels could not be supported on any scale. However, there are two other points we would also have to bear in mind, which were discussed in Chapter 7. First, that in many Third World countries indigenous medical practice has been neglected or restricted, and second, that the influence of the 'world health care system' leads many Third World countries to train health workers or adopt other forms of health care that are not always appropriate to their own needs. In these circumstances it would not be surprising to find at least some countries trying to support secondary and tertiary levels of care that they cannot afford, while neglecting primary care. This is the kind of situation that exists in Ghana, where there is a mismatch between the expenditure on different levels of care and the needs of the population is shown strikingly in Figure 9.3

In short, the financial resources of the nation are being allocated in reverse proportion to the numbers of people in need — a massive 40 per cent of total expenditure is consumed by the tertiary care facilities in the Korle Bu Hospital in the capital, Accra, meeting the needs of only 1 per cent of the population.

Because of inadequate public health and primary care services, patients with preventable conditions overload the hospital services, which leads to greater demand for even more hospital services. As more resources are put into the construction and equipping of hospitals, and the training of sophisticated health workers, fewer and fewer resources are left to develop primary care. The outcome of this process between 1960 and 1977 can be seen in Table 9.1.

Despite a four-fold increase in health care expenditure (in real terms) over this period, the infant mortality rate (IMR) — a sensitive indicator of the health status of a population — remained stubbornly high, and was still 130 per 1 000 live births in 1976. In addition there were large regional inequalities, with the IMR ranging from 63 in the Greater Accra Region on the coast around the capital to 234 in the most northerly region which borders the desert area of the Sahel.

Table 9.1 Health service staffing and facilities in Ghana, 1960–77

Staff/facilities	1960	1977	increase (%)
Doctors	383	1 100	287
Dentists	19	60	216
Nurses	1 554	7 840	405
Hospital beds	5 787	13 500	133

(Source: Morrow, 1983, p.276)

The way in which inappropriate patterns of health care in Third World countries are influenced by industrialised countries with very different health problems can be seen clearly by examining the way in which modern medical techniques 'diffuse' across the world from rich to poor countries. In one study, the economist David Piachaud drew up a list of eight modern medical techniques — four diagnostic and four therapeutic (in intention at least) — to see which had been introduced in Third World countries (Piachaud, 1979). Included among the techniques were laser-beam therapy (capital cost around £35 000–40 000 in 1977), renal dialysis (£10 000 per patient treated in 1977) and computerised tomography (£200 000 capital cost per 'CT' scanner in 1977, plus £50 000 annual running costs). Of the forty countries for which data were made available, twenty-two had introduced five or more of these techniques and almost all had been first introduced in government-financed teaching institutions.

Rather than shifting resources from secondary and tertiary care to primary care, many Third World countries have attempted to distribute the former more widely. Two methods in particular have been used — compulsory rural service and medical camps. *Compulsory rural service* involves forcing doctors and other highly-trained staff to work in hospitals in remote rural areas for a few years after qualifying. Compulsion is almost universally resented by such staff who wish to stay in the capital, specialise, and enjoy both urban life and (in many countries) the profits of the private practice that awaits them. Not only is their training and attitude inappropriate for rural communities, but most of them have rarely set foot outside the urban world of the capital city before. Their resentment at compulsory service is often compounded by the lack of support they receive from their government in the way of supplies and equipment. After two or three years they return home leaving the rural community to await the next conscript.

The second way of distributing secondary and tertiary care more widely is through *medical camps*. These may be organised either internationally or within a country. In the case of the former, industrialised countries send teams of staff and equipment to the Third World for short periods of time to provide relatively specialised, sophisticated care for large numbers of people. For example, ophthalmic surgeons have been sent from Europe to perform hundreds of eye operations in a few weeks.

☐ What historical example of travelling surgeons can you recall?

■ Greek physicians.

Some Third World countries have also established camps within their own country, sending doctors from the main hospital in the capital city to remote rural areas. In Nepal, camps still take place twice a year at the same time as the Royal Court moves away from the capital, Kathmandu. The whole range of medical specialities travels with the King. Tented accommodation is set up and people come from all the surrounding area with health problems which have arisen since the previous camp and which the poorly staffed and equipped local district hospital has been unable to treat.

Although camps may be a highly appropriate way of delivering some specialised services, the experience of this approach has not always been a happy one. The story of sterilisation camps in India in the late 1970s is a worrying example of how the model can be abused. Run by the then Prime Minister, Indira Gandhi, through her son Sanjay, the camps attracted much criticism and contributed to the temporary downfall of her government. The determination with which the camps attained their target number of sterilisations included rewarding people with transistor radios for undergoing the operation.

Vertical and horizontal health programmes

We have seen how useful the primary–secondary–tertiary model can be to tease out patterns of health care access and distribution. We have also seen just how chronic some of

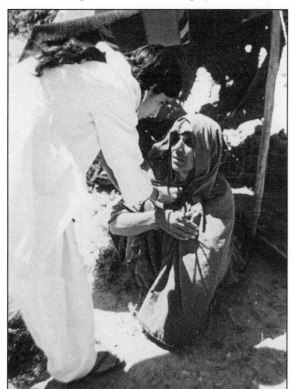

Figure 9.4 An encounter between nomads and travelling doctors in the Sahel, Niger.

the problems of access and distribution can be. Let us now introduce another way of thinking about the organisation of formal health care that focuses not on levels of specialisation but on the organisational approach to tackling health problems.

From this perspective, the two models that we will encounter most frequently are the '*vertical*' health programme and the '*horizontal*' health programme:

> the vertical approach calls for the solution of a given health problem through the application of specific measures through single-purpose machinery ... the horizontal approach seeks to tackle the overall health problems on a wide front and on a long-term basis through the creation of a system of permanent institutions commonly known as 'general health services'. (Gonzalez, 1965, p.2)

☐ What examples of vertical programmes can you recall from previous chapters in the book?

■ Examples include the attempts to control plague and leprosy in medieval Europe, venereal disease in early twentieth-century England, and yellow fever and malaria in Panama.

In fact, vertical programmes frequently have been used in many industrialised countries. Some of the most spectacular examples have been worldwide in scope, the best-known being the eradication of smallpox.* But there have been other less dramatic but highly effective campaigns. In parts of Africa, trypanosomiasis (sleeping sickness), plague and hookworm have been brought under control in this way.

There are two features of vertical programmes that make them particularly appropriate for Third World countries. First, most of the work, such as spraying insecticides, can be largely carried out by unskilled workers. Even the administration of mass vaccination camps can be undertaken by staff with only a few weeks training. Second, their organisational structure, in which the key decision-making is taken by a small central group, is suited to countries in which there are few technical experts such as doctors and epidemiologists. If necessary, experts can be brought from industrialised countries. In addition both Third World governments and external donors and agencies are attracted by the prospect of funding services that are only required for a relatively short time, as is the case, in theory, with disease eradication programmes, rather than making open-ended commitments to fund continuing services.

However, some features of vertical programmes became the focus of criticism in the 1960s and 1970s. First, doubts

were expressed about the programmes' temporary nature. While some vertical programmes included a permanent presence in rural areas, they usually consisted of intermittent, mobile, mass campaigns with no provision for care between visits. Second, the reliance on a small group of 'experts' in the capital cities, or even in a distant country, was a cause for concern. There was little or no consultation with, or involvement of, the local people in villages and towns. This raised the question of who should decide on priorities for health care services — local people, governments, experts, or international agencies — as each group would have different opinions based on their interests. And third, there was concern about the degree to which vertical programmes were dependent on factors external to the country and beyond the country's control.

This is well illustrated by the example of the malaria eradication programme in India. When the campaign started in 1953 there had been around 800 000 deaths a year and about 75 million cases. Largely through house-spraying with residual insecticides, a rapid fall in morbidity and mortality had been achieved so that by 1965 eradication appeared to be within grasp. However, the following year a resurgence in malaria cases began, so that by 1975 there were once again over 5 million cases though only about 100 reported deaths.

Several reasons have been suggested for the resurgence:

> With malaria control almost achieved, crucial and damaging delays occurred in the allotment of foreign exchange to import insecticides and the sense of urgency seems to have been lost through complacency on the part of individual citizens and of Government, central and state, civil servant and politician alike. (Akhtar and Learmonth, 1977, p.69)

The long list of other factors that are thought to have contributed to the resurgence of malaria in India included the cessation of international aid, increases in government

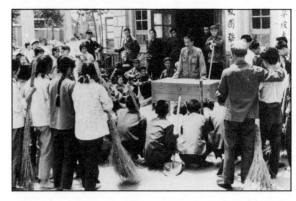

Figure 9.5 A rural Chinese community in the 1960s being addressed at the beginning of a Patriotic Health Campaign.

*The campaign to eradicate smallpox is discussed in *The Biology of Health and Disease, ibid.* (U205 Book IV).

expenditure on defence to meet the perceived military threat posed by China, crop failures resulting in increased spending on food imports, an increased resistance of mosquitoes to the insecticides being used, and the closure of the Suez Canal, arising out of the Middle East War of 1967, which prevented supplies of insecticides reaching India.

The vulnerability of vertical programmes in Third World countries which are dependent on external aid, technology and professional support was underlined by the relative successes that were achieved in China during the 1950s. While the Chinese, like other Third World governments, adopted vertical programmes, they did so by involving their own people rather than relying on the industrialised world. This is a striking example of how patterns of health care reflect the wider social and political structures of a country.

In 1949 in China the communists, led by Mao Tse Tung and with the support of the peasants who constituted the great majority of the population, had gained power. During the period 1950 to 1952 the central objective of Chinese policy was the economic rehabilitation of the country after years of war and occupation. This objective was reflected in the health policies of the period: the establishment of a basic health care organisation and the launching of a campaign to eradicate the main infectious and parasitic diseases. This involved dispersing medical care from the heavily concentrated urban bases to the rural population by establishing health teams. The early work of the teams focused on the prevention of epidemics, setting up maternal and child health services and training local people in their own villages to carry out such activities as vaccinations.

Part of the labour force necessary for this strategy was created by the use of auxiliary workers under the supervision of the 20 000 doctors in the country who had been trained in western medicine. The work of the health teams was not conducted in isolation from the rest of the population, however. From 1952, mass campaigns, or 'Patriotic Health Campaigns', were launched, in which virtually the entire population was enlisted to eliminate contaminated water supplies, improve sanitation, and eradicate the 'four pests': rats, mosquitoes, bedbugs and flies.

The reduction in mortality from some infectious diseases during the early 1950s is shown in Table 9.2.

Some other factors should also be taken into account when considering the figures above. In the years from 1936 to 1950 China had been torn apart by Japanese invasion and by civil war. The cessation of fighting and the return to some sort of order would in itself have led to a fall in mortality rates in the early 1950s.

With the benefit of hindsight, it is also necessary to raise a caution against the accuracy of these statistics: it is now known that in the later 1950s — during the 'Great Leap Forward' — many basic demographic statistics were not collected, although 'figures' continued to be published. The IMR of 34 in 1956, for example, quoted in the table and the article from which it was drawn, is frankly unbelievable. In 1984 the officially reported rates were 165 for 1960, and 67 by 1982. Nevertheless, the achievements of the government, and not least the people, during that period cannot be dismissed.

Another example of the effectiveness of Chinese policies was the campaign in the late 1950s and 1960s to eliminate schistosomiasis.* The campaign was directed at the elimination of the intermediate host — snails — by laboriously, temporarily draining infested ditches, pools, canals and streams, and removing their chief habitat — the top three inches of mud at the sides. As Joshua Horn (an English surgeon who worked in China during this period) pointed out, this policy

> could not possibly succeed without the leadership of the Party, without the fullest and most active support from millions of people, and without a correct overall strategic plan. (Horn, 1969, p.96)

*The natural history and life-cycle of schistosomiasis is described in *The Health of Nations, ibid.* (U205 Book III).

Table 9.2 Changes in mortality rate in China, 1950–1956.

Disease/Group	Mortality rate (per 000) in		Percentage reduction 1950–1956
	1950	1956	
Measles	86.0	16.5	81
Dysentry	38.0	4.7	88
Scarlet fever	78.0	16.8	79
Infant mortality	117.0	34.0	71
Overall mortality	17.0	11.4	33

(Source: Rifkin and Kaplinsky, 1973, Table 1, p.221)

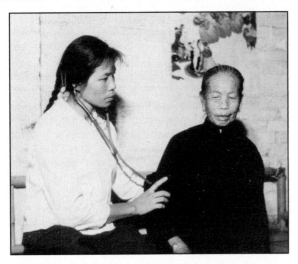

Figure 9.6 A barefoot doctor at work in the Ping Chou commune, China.

The tactics drew heavily on the political and military tactics used during the revolutionary war:

> ... Mao Tse Tung summarized a set of military tactics which, within two years, helped to win nation-wide victory. One of them was — In every battle, concentrate an absolutely superior force, encircle the enemy forces completely, strive to wipe them out thoroughly and do not let any escape from the net! This tactic was applied in the battle against the snails by selecting focal points for decisive attack. Of the ten infected counties around Shanghai, two were selected as the main targets in the early stages of what was to be a prolonged campaign. All available labour power, medical resources, pumps, river-draining and damming equipment were concentrated in these two counties and, within a short time, the snails there had suffered a mortal blow. Then the forces were regrouped and the attack was directed elsewhere. Gradually, extensive snail-free zones were created. (Horn, 1969, p.97)

This military analogy extended to 'snail-sweeps', 'anti-snail patrols', and 'snail-spotters'. By the late 1960s, the campaign against schistosomiasis had still not completely eliminated the disease, but the length of river banks infected had reportedly been cut from 4.3 million metres to 65 thousand metres, and cases of human infection and mortality greatly reduced.

☐ Reflecting on what has been said above of Chinese health care, how do you think it fits the vertical/horizontal models?

■ Chinese health care programmes in the 1950s and 1960s contained elements of both: there were con-

centrated campaigns against specific diseases, but also the establishment of more general, 'horizontal' health services, such as health teams and the training of auxiliary workers.

The problems experienced by vertical health programmes elsewhere, and the general acclaim with which the Chinese experience was met, led in the 1960s and 1970s to an increasing emphasis on the need for horizontal programmes as the only way to tackle effectively the disease problems of Third World countries. And just as the earlier vertical programmes adopted by national governments had been encouraged and aided by international organisations, and in particular the World Health Organization, so the move towards horizontal programmes was also promoted by the WHO.

Before looking at the practical achievements and problems of this change in direction, it is worth looking briefly at a document issued by the WHO in 1978 that summarised the policy: the *Declaration of Alma-Ata*, published in 1978 as the outcome of an international conference held in the capital city of Kazakhstan in the USSR. Like all such WHO documents, the *Declaration of Alma-Ata* represented the end result of an extremely long and complex process of consultation and negotiation with representatives of all member-countries that wished to state a point of view. As such it was a diplomatically agreed statement of general intent rather than a plan.

Adopted by the WHO under the slogan 'Health for All by the year 2000', the document declared that health was a fundamental human right and that existing inequalities in health status between people was unacceptable. While recognising that much of the inequalities arose from the international economic order which favoured some countries and harmed others, it considered that the provision of adequate health care was a basic responsibility of all governments, and that the key to attaining health for all by the year 2000 was a horizontal programme of health care based on primary care.

A central feature of the Declaration was recognition of the need for health services to be integrated at four different levels: vertical programmes were to be combined in a multi-purpose horizontal programme which encompassed both preventive and curative activities; primary health care was to be integrated with the local community it was serving, rather than implanted and largely controlled from outside by a central authority; health care was to be integrated with other aspects of development: improvements in food production, provision of a clean water supply, the establishment of local industries to meet many basic needs, and land reform; and modern medicine was to be integrated with traditional indigenous medicine.

☐ In light of earlier discussion, why do you think the

emphasis was placed on the *primary* level of care?

■ Secondary and tertiary levels of care are expensive to provide and only cater for a small proportion of the health care needs of Third World countries.

Other aspects of the document also drew on past experience. For example the recognition that wider forms of development were important to the promotion of health stemmed in part from the experiences of places such as Kerala State in the south-west tip of India. Since its formation in 1956, Kerala has pursued policies of income redistribution through reform of the land tenure system, employment security, free education at primary level, and some redistribution of health resources away from urban areas. Despite the relative poverty of Kerala compared with some other Indian states (such as Punjab and Maharashtra), by 1981 the people of Kerala had higher literacy rates than any other state, life expectancy at birth was 63.8 years compared to 52 years for the whole country, and the infant mortality rate was 55 per 1000 births compared to 125 for all India. And yet during the period the per capita expenditure on formal health services was less than the average for all India.

The Alma-Ata Declaration also reaffirmed the view that health care at the primary care level could be provided by people other than doctors. Again this was based on a number of previous experiences, and in particular the auxiliary workers and barefoot doctors that had been introduced in China. Let's take a closer look at these *village health workers*.

Despite variations of detail between countries, village health workers all share the same basic objectives. With minimal training, they live in the communities they serve and using locally available materials attempt to improve the villagers' health through preventive, rather than curative, measures. Typical activities include encouraging the construction of pit latrines (simply holes in the ground covered by a shelter) and the boiling of all drinking water.

Another key aspect of their work is to maximise community participation in undertaking such measures. (One of the major criticisms that had been made of the vertical programmes was that they engendered dependency because there was often little or no local involvement. For example, insecticide sprayers would turn up every few months and spray the houses to combat mosquitoes, but in the intervening periods no action was taken by local people.) Both the benefits and the problems associated with village health workers are discussed in an article by David Werner in the Course Reader* and you should now read it.

* Werner, D., 'The village health worker — lackey or liberator?', in Black, N., *et al.* (eds), *ibid.*

□ Werner describes two main patterns of provision of primary care workers in the Third World — village health workers and auxiliary nurses/health workers. What aspects of the former does Werner consider to be advantageous?

■ They usually require a shorter training period; they are selected *from* the community in which they will work; they may be paid by the local people.

□ What does Werner consider to be the underlying cause of disease?

■ Inequality — of health, of land, of educational opportunity, of political representation and of basic human rights.

□ In what way does Werner consider village health workers can improve people's health?

■ Some palliation can be achieved through simple curative and preventive work such as encouraging the building of pit latrines. However, major change can only be brought about by educating people about the wider political factors that lead to their poor health — the role of village worker as liberator.

As we saw, the Alma-Ata Declaration also acknowledges the importance of wider aspects of economic and social change. But to what extent is it feasible to consider changing the socio-economic order of a country *by means of* primary health care? As Werner himself points out, 'the politico-economic structure of the country must necessarily influence the extent to which its rural health program is community-supportive or not'. In other words, a country's health care system will be moulded by the wider social structure, rather than the other way round.

In the absence of such socio-economic changes, critics of the Declaration have suggested that its slogan should be at most the more limited 'Health *care* for all'. In addition, they have pointed out that the primary health care approach requires people to change their behaviour in ways that often seem inappropriate to them, and imposes costs on them that are seldom taken into account. David Nabarro, a British doctor who has been actively involved in primary health care services, has described an example of the sorts of difficulties that can arise:

In rural areas of India, severe disease is most common during the early monsoon months while family members are particularly busy in the fields. Time is precious — families may well consider that an hour or two away from the fields will have an adverse effect on the subsequent harvest. Yet it is spare time, more than anything, which is needed by parents when nursing a sick child through a bad attack of diarrhoea — time to encourage the child to eat or drink, and time to attend a clinic to receive treatment and medical advice. During the months when they and their children are most likely to be ill, poor farmers and agricultural labourers are so short of time, food and cash they are unlikely to adopt new measures which will prevent or contain illness. (Nabarro, 1982, pp.6–7)

These problems in trying to create effective primary health care systems highlight one of the themes of this book: that health care is located firmly in a much wider social context, and parts of it — for example, the Chinese version of the village health worker — cannot simply be lifted out of their original context and transplanted. As we noted at the end of Chapter 7, this wider context can be taken to include not just the immediate social environment of all the activities that comprise caring for health, but also a long historical process that has led at present to a gap — indeed a gulf — that separates the world into a small group of industrialised countries and a very much larger group of countries that so far have not industrialised. Finding appropriate ways of organising health care is a vitally important task, but it is also just one aspect of a very much bigger task, which is to bridge this global gap.

In 1983 the WHO produced an assessment of progress in the 'march towards Health for All'. Discussing this assessment in an interview in 1983, the WHO director responsible for coordinating the entire 'Health for All' strategy was asked whether access to primary health care had generally improved over the previous five years: 'Probably not, taking the world as a whole. In certain countries, yes. But because the population increase has been greatest in those areas where there has been no development in primary health care, we are probably rather worse off now than we were five years ago'. Asked whether he had cause to regret the slogan 'Health for All by the year 2000', Dr Hellberg replied 'No, I don't. If you look at any sector or any planning exercise, the year 2000 is used. The important thing is that it forces people to look forward, providing a prospective view. In the past, the whole medical and health system had a retrospective view, reacting to what had already happened. Sometimes I am surprised at how well it works in this respect. Its forward look is its main emphasis, just as the words Liberty, Equality, Fraternity were during the French Revolution.' And finally, when will we achieve Health for All? 'In some ways you can say, perhaps never. Some countries will achieve the goals they have put for their population by the year 2000. But the really tough goal of having a reasonable level of health and well-being so that everyone on the planet can live a decent human life — I dare not predict when that can take place' (Hellberg, 1983, pp.10 and 12).

Objectives for Chapter 9

When you have finished studying this chapter, you should be able to:

9.1 Explain what is meant by primary, secondary, and tertiary care, and describe some of the diverse ways that health care is organised in industrial countries.

9.2 Explain what is meant by vertical and by horizontal programmes, and their respective advantages and disadvantages as models for the delivery of health care in the Third World.

Questions for Chapter 9

1 (*Objective 9.1*) In Chapter 4 we discussed the Dawson Report, published in Britain in 1920. How did it fit into the primary/secondary/tertiary model?

2 (*Objective 9.2*) In the discussion of vertical health programmes in Third World countries, the problem of dependency arose in two different contexts. What were they?

10
Thinking about health care

We began this book with an argument that in order to understand health care it is insufficient to concentrate on the formal health sector, in one country, in the present, and is instead necessary to take a broad sweep through time and space, exploring the many different human activities that fit the description 'caring for health' — their historical development, and the extent to which they vary from one society to another.

This argument has been at the very heart of the entire book, directing the kind of evidence we decided to include, and guiding the interpretations we placed on it. If the reader at this point is still neither convinced that a great deal of care is provided outside the formal health care sector, nor that health care is influenced in all manner of ways by its social and economic context, nor that our perception of the present can be altered by our awareness of the past, then she or he is not going to be persuaded by a few words in a concluding chapter, for the argument rests largely on the evidence.

Yet that is not quite the end of the story. To be sure, if we were interested only in expanding our understanding of health care, if we were to adopt the contemplative stance advocated in Montaigne's statement 'others shape the man; I portray him', then we could conclude the argument of the book along the lines 'there it rests, let it lie'. But most of us want to do more than this. In our own ways, and for our own reasons, most of us want to put our knowledge to some use. We want to contemplate in order that we can prescribe action; in short, we want not just to understand the world but to change it, or at least our own little corner of it.

We must conclude therefore with another argument. This book has been in part a preparation, a terrain which we think has had to be traversed before it is possible to confront head-on the dilemmas of and prospects for contemporary health care. These dilemmas and prospects all concern *policy*, that is, the possibilities for *consciously directed change*. As we look back on history and diversity, therefore, what lessons can we learn that might cast light on these issues?

What is health care?

Let's first briefly review some of the basic messages of the book. As we have seen, health care is an expression that covers many different activities.

☐ List some examples of the range of activities, people and topics to which the term 'health care' can be applied.

■ The term includes not just direct medical treatment but far broader matters such as conditions of employment or the control of waste; it ranges from a consultation with a doctor to a national or even a global health service; it covers personal hygiene as well as public health; and it consists both of women at home nursing elderly relatives and specialists in modern teaching hospitals who never actually see a patient.

All of these can be lumped together under the broad heading of health care. We can therefore talk of a caring individual and, if we like, of a caring society. And indeed we can even try to compare the extent to which different societies do care about health.

☐ What criteria might be used to do this in contemporary societies?

■ Some of the more frequently used are: the proportion of national income spent on health care; the distribution of health care across, for example, class, gender, or region; and rates of morbidity, disability and mortality.

However, partly because of the sheer range of activities that can be called health care, none of these measures will do by itself. Two countries may spend similar amounts on their formal health care sector, but very different amounts on the provision of water, sewage and sanitation services. Or a country may have a very small formal health care sector but an elaborate and highly developed pattern of lay care. The *range* of activities must always be kept in mind, for it reaches into every level and every part of human society. This is the first lesson of the book.

The problem of trying to decide how much an individual or society cares about health, however, does not stem only from the range of activities that have to be taken into account. Consider, for example, the following question.

☐ Is Britain a more caring society as regards health than it was five or six hundred years ago?

■ Formal health care services have been expanded, do some new things, and are far more widely available. There has also been a huge decline in mortality rates, though it is not entirely clear how much of this improvement can be attributed to health care. There must also be some doubts about the caring nature of some health services. What sort of care can be provided by large, often impersonal organisations? Is caring the same when it is done for a living, rather than as a part of family responsibilities?

The fact is that grouping a wide range of activities together under the heading 'health care' begs the question whether 'care' is quite the right word, and whether health is the primary purpose. Institutional care, for example, has been subject to repeated criticism, from the French revolutionary St Just's attack upon hospitals to the critique of large traditional mental hospitals mounted in the 1960s.* The grounds for such criticisms have often been precisely that inmates or patients are not being 'cared' for in any conventional sense of the word. So what is the nature of such forms of care, that may force people to be 'cared' for and deny them the opportunity to decide whether or not to accept?

To answer this question, let's look more closely at the motives that prompt people to provide health care for others, both formally and informally. Closest to what is normally meant by 'care' is the notion that care is either a duty, or a right, or else it is a matter of sentiment, a fellow-feeling: to relieve the suffering of others, diagnose their ills and help guard them against future ailments.

☐ List examples of such caring motives from the rest of the book.

■ You might have mentioned some of the motives behind religious hospitals, the founding of voluntary hospitals and dispensaries, the humanitarian attempts

to reform asylums, the granting of bequests and alms for the poor. There are also the attempts to develop formal health services for all, and more equal distribution of services. And finally, there is the enormous amount of health care that is prompted by the ties of love and obligation within the family, and by feelings of affection and professional duty amongst paid carers.

Such caring motives, however, are not the only ones. Indeed, whereas religions, governments, professions and families may all prefer to have their motives described in this fashion, many of their actions could be interpreted differently: as motivated by self-interest.

☐ Why might self-interest prompt religions, governments, employers, health occupations or families to provide health care?

■ Health care might win religions both new converts and new bequests; it might offer governments a way of heading off social unrest, winning elections, or preparing for war — making the nation 'fighting fit'. To employers it might create a more productive and more loyal work force; to medical practitioners more health care might mean more job opportunities, more income, or more status; to families and friends it might be a loan-in-kind, to be repaid when they themselves are in need.

So, if the first lesson of the book is the extraordinary range of health care, the ambiguity of motive and purpose that surrounds that care is the second basic lesson — the reasons why it exists may be as varied as the forms that it takes.

What are the policy questions?

Having summarised these fundamental lessons, let us now turn to consider *policy*. With a subject as complex as health care, it is always easy to draw up a list of '*the* issues'; but more difficult to get even two people to agree on the same list. Let's plunge straight in by proposing a series of issues that seem to dominate a great deal of contemporary policy, analysis, research and debate. First, there is the *effectiveness* of health care; second, its *cost*; third, *control and decision-making*; fourth, *civil liberties* and personal rights; and finally, distribution, access, and *equality*. The list probably omits things some people would have included, and includes things others would have left out, but it is a starting point that allows us to address a variety of topics.

The first is *effectiveness*. It is often pointed out that many forms of health care often seem to have had no discernible impact on health, that until the late nineteenth century medicine had a very limited range of demonstrably effective treatments on offer, and that even now the amount of formal health care an industrialised country supports bears little relation to the healthiness of its population.

*A much lengthier examination of the problems of institutional care is given in *Experiencing and Explaining Disease, ibid.*, Chapter 13 (U205 Book VI).

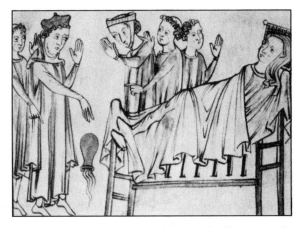

Figure 10.1 Effectiveness: an age-old issue. This illustration of a sick lady with her physician is from a thirteenth-century text ascribed to Constantine the African. The dropped urine flask (and the attitudes of those present) indicate that the case is hopeless.

☐ What reasons can you think of for the existence of health care when it is often, apparently, so ineffective?

■ There would seem to be at least three distinct reasons. The first and perhaps most important is that for all the body's extraordinary defensive and recuperative powers it still remains vulnerable in many different ways. We are all mortal, much of the time most of us would like to be happy and fit as well as alive. Achieving all these simultaneously can be very hard — yet we all nurture the hope that it is possible. A great deal of health care is based on this hope: hope that if we brush our teeth every day we will have no need for dentures; the hope that if only we could find the right doctor then surely we would be cured. The second reason, as you have seen, is that other people share our hopes. They too, for reasons of charity, religion, human solidarity or professional duty wish us well; they too hope. And the third reason is that health care is not just about saving lives and curing illness. As you have seen, there are many other motives for providing it.

There is therefore a major discrepancy between the enormous human desire for health care — a desire fed by many different streams — and the reality of what health care provides. There is also the possibility that a type of health care that is very ineffective by one set of criteria may be very effective according to another. The concentration of a Third World country's formal health care resources on a single teaching hospital in the capital city may be a very ineffective way of improving the health of a largely rural population, but a very effective way for the government to stay in favour with its urban supporters. Policies to improve effectiveness are not therefore simply about choosing

between different ways of attaining the same objective, although that is part of it; they are also about choosing objectives themselves, and recognising that not everyone will agree with those objectives.

A second recurring issue in health care is that of *cost*. One strand of concern over cost, predominant in contemporary debate in industrialised countries, is that the formal health care sector costs too much to provide.

☐ What previous instances of concern over the cost of formal health care can you recollect?

■ The Poor Law Amendment Act of 1834 was introduced in response to the rising costs of providing poor relief. We also saw that some of the medieval hospitals of London were strongly criticised for being extravagant.

But once it has been acknowledged that the formal health care sector represents but a small part of all caring for health, then it must also be accepted that the costs of the formal health care sector represent but a small part of the total cost of caring for health: many other costs are incurred by families, friends and relatives, by patients themselves, by employers or public authorities. And trying to reduce costs in one area, such as institutional care, may result, for example, in increasing costs for lay carers. Some caution is required, therefore, to avoid arbitrarily including some costs and excluding others.

Why should cost recur time and again as a health care issue? The first reason is linked to that of effectiveness, to getting value for money out of health care, for there are always doubts about whether health care is having the effects claimed for it. There are also always other competing uses to which health care resources can be put: for example, the Elizabethan government cast covetous eyes on the church revenues used to support monastic hospitals, seeing instead a way of bolstering state income that could finance other things such as an expanded navy. And finally, there is the notion of the *sick role* — the idea that sickness is not an absolute condition but a relative social state, a permitted form of social deviance.

☐ How might the concept of the sick role relate to concern over the cost of health care?

■ Every society faces the problem of deciding how many people it can *afford* to sustain in the sick role, whether it be a group of gatherer-hunters, a small medieval village, or a contemporary industrialised state. Cost is therefore closely bound up with the very way in which people are defined as sick or not, and what rights they receive.

If such decisions have to be made, and if sickness and the right to formal health care has to be continually defined and redefined, how and by whom are such decisions made? For such reasons the issue of *control and decision making* repays examination in any society's health care activities, and again is central to contemporary debates on policy.

☐ List some of the different people and groups who have been at some time involved in controlling formal health care.

■ Central government, local government, religions, political parties, insurance companies, the medical profession, charities, commercial enterprises, and men.

As this list suggests, at any one time several different groups are each trying to exert some control — control over other groups, over particular aspects of health care, or over their own position.

Sometimes, control and decision making are manifested in obvious and direct ways: the control exercised by a profession through a register of practitioners, or the decisions of a government department over the ownership of hospitals. But control and decision making can take many different forms.

☐ For example, recall the prevailing social and economic policy in early nineteenth-century England, and what it seemed to imply for central government control and decision making.

■ The policy was *laissez-faire*, or 'leave well alone'. It implied that the government would not actively try to control things, but would simply leave decision making to individuals and markets.

The *laissez-faire* conception of a decision-making mechanism is not that of an hierarchical authority explicitly arriving at decisions and then implementing them; rather, it is an impersonal and indirect mechanism of market transactions. The classic statement of this view was made by Adam Smith in the eighteenth century: the market could be seen as an 'invisible hand' guiding the actions of individuals towards the goal of the good of all society, although the mainspring of individual action was not the good of all, but rather the pursuit of self-interest.

It is not from the benevolence of the butcher, the brewer or the baker, that we expect our dinner, but from their regard to their own interest. We address ourselves, not to their humanity, but to their self-love, and never talk to them of our own necessities, but of their advantages. Nobody but a beggar chooses to depend chiefly upon the benevolence of his fellow-citizens. (Smith, 1976 edition, pp.26–7)

By the same token, the 'decision' to provide a hospital or water-supply could be left to the market. However, if we stay with the example of the *laissez-faire* policies of early nineteenth-century England, we might recall the disparity between theory and practice. In practice, non-

interventionist policies were pursued by systematic and growing involvement of government not only in health care but in many other areas. Walking from Westminster Bridge to Trafalgar Square, one might wryly observe that almost all the government buildings that are passed, from the Houses of Parliament to the far end of Whitehall, were enlarged or built in the high years of *laissez-faire*. Policy and practice are often very different, and when the object of policy is something as complex as health care, something that reaches into almost every nook and cranny of society, then policies on the control of one area may have unforeseen or unintended ramifications in other areas.

Some of the further issues in our list arose as a popular rallying call only late in our history of health care, though they have since exerted an immense influence: *liberty, equality and fraternity* — though we might substitute 'fellowship' or 'solidarity' for the last, so that women as well as men are included.

☐ How might *liberty* arise as an issue in health care?

■ First, the provision of health care may — as in the case of some inmates in mental illness or quarantine hospitals — result in the denial of personal liberty. Other issues include the liberty of medical practitioners to exercise their clinical freedom, and whether restriction of this freedom is a curtailment of their own and their patients' liberties; the liberty of the individual to sue doctors or to pollute others' environment or to opt out of public health measures such as fluoridation of water; the notion that health care is a *right*, and that lack of access to it is a denial of liberty; the question of whether legal restrictions on abortion, contraception, dissection or euthanasia maintain or suppress liberties; and finally, whether individuals should be at complete liberty to choose their medical practitioners, or whether such liberty should be restricted via state licensing, or by formal referral systems, and so forth.

Just as there are many debates over liberty, so *equality* — or its lack — has also been a major focus of interest. Historically, institutional forms of health care have been intimately associated with social provision for the poor: medical relief and poor relief have often been inseparable. And because poor relief has often been provided by public bodies that have been obliged to keep records, accounts and reports for reasons of public accountability, so there sometimes exists a lot more information about health care for the poor than for the rich. But in all cases, past and present, enough information exists for us to know that the pursuit of equality — however defined — in the provision of health care is a course strewn with obstacles. One of these is that equality and liberty may be in conflict: equality of access to health care, for example, may be seen as an infringement of the liberty to spend money obtaining additional health care.

☐ Health care raises issues of equality not only in the distribution of access to care, however. What other aspect of inequality has recurred throughout the book?
■ Perhaps the most important is the deep-rooted *gender* inequality among health carers.

The primary responsibility for providing lay health care is typically ascribed to women. And in formal health care, although men predominate in the senior posts of medicine, women are the largest group of workers. Moreover, this picture is far from new: in ancient Greece women were entirely excluded from doctoring and where women have engaged in medical practice there have often been serious attempts to exclude them. Even in midwifery, the one area traditionally reserved for women, male obstetricians have come to dominate the scene (to the extent even of rendering midwifery illegal in some parts of the USA).

In the account of health care that this book has provided, the persistence and ramifications of gender inequalities have been recurring themes. Yet it is unlikely that the subject would have appeared had we been writing this book fifty or even twenty years ago, and it is apparent from many of the older quotations in the book that until very recently 'man' was used to mean 'human' and 'he' to denote 'she' also. And only in recent years has the gender content of words such as 'fraternity' become an issue to a large number of people. All of which illustrates that history is not a fixed body of knowledge, but rather is the way in which the present looks at the past and tries to interpret it in the light of contemporary concerns and contemporary ways of thinking.

History and diversity: taking leave
So how has this book looked at the past, and what contemporary ways of thinking are reflected in it? The emphasis has been on assembling empirical data on aspects of health care, but that still implies some choice of what to include and what to leave out, and that in turn implies some theoretical view of the world. What is it?

As we have seen, changing beliefs, ideas, customs, religions, institutions and material circumstances are all eventually reflected in one way or another in health care. What causes all these extraordinary changes in human society is a question to which a variety of answers are on offer.

One view places a great deal of emphasis on the power of ideas, thought, knowledge, intellect and theory. Some of these — for example, miasmic theory — have fundamentally influenced health care. On this account, 'wrong' ideas and 'right' ideas can be equally powerful, and may exert their greatest force on people hardly aware that they hold them: 'Practical men', wrote John Maynard Keynes (one of the twentieth century's most influential economic theorists),

> who believe themselves to be quite exempt from any intellectual influences, are usually the slaves of some defunct economist. Madmen in authority, who hear voices in the air, are distilling their frenzy from some academic scribbler of a few years back. (Keynes, 1936, Chapter 24, v)

The most powerful 'idea' to appear in the book, however, was not the work of any individual 'scribbler' but the collective creation of many men and women over a very long period of time: science and the *scientific method*. The medical system that was transformed by the use of the scientific method we have referred to as *modern medicine* — not western medicine because it is not owned and was not solely created by the west, and not scientific medicine because much of it is still not scientific. None the less, modern medicine is more science-based than any other system, and this is part of the reason why it continues to spread around the world.

But set against this, there is another view, that places much more emphasis on the material conditions of life, and sees most features of society, including ideas, as traceable to the basic way in which the production of subsistence and wealth is organised in a society. On this account, the fundamental characteristics of health care over the period we have surveyed depends on whether that society was a slave society, a feudal society or a capitalist society, for as each replaced its predecessor so new forms of health care, of ideas and thought, of family, religion, law and education, replaced the old forms. The classic formulation of this view was by Marx and Engels:

> ... the class which is the ruling *material* force of society, is at the same time its ruling intellectual force. The class which has the means of material production at its disposal, has control at the same time over the means of mental production. (Marx and Engels, 1965 edition, p.60)

There are other theories, too, that have sought to organise all facets of history and social change around a single factor, whether this be the inescapable presence of disease or some spiritual vision held by a civilisation. Can we make a choice between them, or — perhaps a more appropriate question — do we have to?

All such theories can be seen as attempts to produce a 'total history', that is, a history that tries to relate all phenomena to one single causal centre: ideas, class conflict or whatever. Once a causal centre has been chosen, the next step is to attempt to trace its effect in all aspects and levels of society: social, religious, political, economic and legal, and in health care, education, entertainment, welfare and warfare. Underlying this book, however, there is no single causal centre, no theory that health care can be explained by reference to one solitary process. Let's recall briefly a concrete example, the discovery of the vectors of transmission of a group of 'tropical' diseases around the turn of this century: the intellectual breakthrough helped make possible giant commercial and economic projects, such as the Panama Canal. At the same time, however, it was in part because of the global expansion of the colonial empires of Europe and North America that tropical disease suddenly became a problem for which it was pressingly important to find a solution. So one theory stressing the importance of ideas and another stressing material circumstances both contain some of the truth, but neither contains all of it; explanations must be sought in several directions at once.

This wider view of history and diversity, summed up in the phrase of the historian, Fernand Braudel, that 'we must think of everything in the plural', comes closest to this book's 'theory'. And when we turn to a closer analysis of the dilemmas of and prospects for contemporary health care, this 'thinking in the plural' must be continued. From the vantage point of this book, it should be possible to view contemporary issues from a number of directions.* But it should also be possible to see that there is no unchanging and universal list of 'issues', any more than there is only one way of thinking about them. Contemporary concerns about health care in Britain may seem as curious and partial to observers elsewhere or in the future as the concerns of our predecessors or of other societies sometimes seem to us. On that note, we have reached the end of one book, but also the beginning of another.

---

*Caring for Health: Dilemmas and Prospects, ibid. (U205 Book VIII), picks up and continues many of the themes of this book.

References
and
further
reading

References

ABEL-SMITH, B. (1960) *A History of the Nursing Profession*, Heinemann.

ABEL-SMITH, B. (1964) *The Hospitals, 1800–1948*, Heinemann.

ABEL-SMITH, B. (1975) *Value for Money in Health Services*, Heinemann.

ABEL-SMITH, B. and MAYNARD, A. (1978) *The Organization, Financing and Cost of Health Care in the EEC*, Commission of the European Communities, SEC(78).2862, Brussels.

ABEL-SMITH, B. and TITMUSS, R. (1954) *The Cost of the National Health Service in England and Wales*, HMSO.

AKHTAR, R. and LEARMONTH, A. (1977) The Resurgence of Malaria in India 1965–1976, *Geojournal*, 1 (5), pp. 69–80.

ALLDERIDGE, P. (1979) Hospitals, Madhouses and Asylums: Cycles in the Care of the Insane, *British Journal of Psychiatry*, 134, pp. 321–334.

ARMENGAUD, A. (1976) Population in Europe, 1700–1914, in C.M. Cipolla (ed.) *The Industrial Revolution 1700–1914*, Harvester.

ASHTON, T.R. (1960) *An Economic History of England: 1870–1939*, Methuen.

BARRACLOUGH, G. (ed.) (1984) *The Times Atlas of World History*, Times Books.

BASCH, P. (1978) *International Health*, Oxford University Press.

BLACK, N., BOSWELL, D., GRAY, A., MURPHY, S. and POPAY, J. (eds) (1984) *Health and Disease: A Reader*, Open University Press. The Course Reader.

BOSTON WOMEN'S HEALTH BOOK COLLECTIVE (1971) *Our Bodies, Ourselves* [British edition, A. Phillips and J.Rakusen (eds) (1979) Penguin].

BRAUDEL, F. (1982) *Civilisation and Capitalism, 15th–18th Century: the Wheels of Commerce*, Collins.

BREARLEY, R. (1984) Medicine in the European Communities, *British Medical Journal*, 288, pp. 1360–1363.

BROCKINGTON, C.F. (1975) *World Health*, 3rd edn, Churchill Livingstone.

BROTHERSTON, J. (1971) Evolution of Medical Practice, in G. McLachlan and T. McKeown (eds) *Medical History and Medical Care*, Oxford University Press.

BRUCE, M. (1968) *The Coming of the Welfare State*, Batsford.

BUER, M.C. (1926) *Health, Wealth and Population, 1760–1815*, George Routledge.

BUNKER, J.P., BARNES, B.A. and MOSTELLER, F. (1977) *Costs, Risks and Benefits of Surgery*, Oxford University Press, New York.

CALDER, A. (1971) *The People's War: Britain 1939–45*, Granada.

CARPENTER, G. (1984) National Health Insurance: a Case Study in the Use of Private Non-Profit Making Organisations in the Provision of Welfare Benefits, *Public Administration*, 62, pp. 71–89.

CASSEDY, J. (1977) Why Self-Help? Americans Alone with their Disease 1880–1950, in G. Risse, R. Numbers and J. Learniff (eds) *Medicine Without Doctors*, Science History Publications, New York.

CHRIST, K. (1984) *The Romans*, Chatto and Windus.

CIPFA (Chartered Institute of Public Finance and Accountancy) (1984) *Health Care UK 1984*, CIPFA.

CIPOLLA, C.M. (ed.) (1972) *The Middle Ages*, Fontana.

CIPOLLA, C.M. (ed.) (1976a) *The Industrial Revolution 1700–1914*, Harvester.

CIPOLLA, C. M. (1976b) *Public Health and the Medical Profession in the Renaissance*, Cambridge University Press.

COCHRANE, A.S., ST LEGER, R. and MOORE, F. (1978) Health Service 'Input' and Mortality 'Output' in Developed Countries, *Journal of Epidemiology and Community Health*, 32, pp. 200–205.

COLLINGS, J.S. (1950) General Practice in England Today:

A Reconnaissance, *Lancet*, **I**, pp. 555–585.

CULLEN, C. (1983) Chinese Science, in P. Corsi and P. Weindling (eds) *Information Sources in the History of Science and Medicine*, Butterworth.

DEANE, P. and COLE, W.A. (1978) *British Economic Growth 1688–1959*, 2nd edn, Cambridge University Press.

DHSS (1980) *Evidence to the National Insurance Advisory Committee*, DHSS.

DICKENS, C. (1844) *Martin Chuzzlewit*, Penguin edn (1970).

DOYLE, W. (1978) *The Old European Order 1660–1800*, Oxford University Press.

DUBOS, R. (1979) The Mirage of Health, in Black, N. *et al.* (1984); *ibid*.

DUNNELL, D. and CARTWRIGHT, A. (1972) *Medicine Takers, Prescribers and Hoarders*, Routledge and Kegan Paul.

ECKSTEIN, H. (1958) *The English Health Service*, Oxford University Press.

ELLIOT-BINNS, C. (1973) The First Form of Care: Analysis of Lay Medicine, *Journal of the Royal College of General Practitioners*, **23**, pp. 255–264.

EVANS, R.G. (1974) Supplier-Induced Demand; some Empirical Evidence and Implications, in M. Perlman (ed.) *The Economics of Health and Medical Care*, pp. 162–173, Macmillan for the International Economics Association.

FARRANT, W. and RUSSELL, J. (1985) *Beating Heart Disease: a Case-Study in the Production of Health Education Material*, Bedford Way Paper, University of London.

FINCH, J. and GROVES, D. (eds) (1983) *A Labour of Love: Women, Work, and Caring*, Routledge and Kegan Paul.

FORSYTH, G. (1966) *Doctors and State Medicine*, Pitman.

FOUCAULT, M. (1973) *Madness and Civilisation*, Vintage Books.

FOUCAULT, M. (1976) *The Birth of the Clinic*, Tavistock.

FRASER, W.H. (1981) *The Coming of the Mass Market, 1850–1914*, Macmillan.

FREIDSON, E. (1960) Client Control and Medical Practice, *American Journal of Sociology*, **65**, pp. 374–382.

GONZALEZ, C.L. (1965) *Mass Campaigns and General Health Services*, Public Health Paper no. 29, WHO, Geneva.

GOODY, J. (1983) *The Development of the Family and Marriage in Europe*, Cambridge University Press.

HACKING, I. (1984) *The Emergence of Probability: a Philosophical Study of Early Ideas about Probability, Induction and Statistical Evidence*, Cambridge University Press.

HALEY, B. (1978) *The Healthy Body and Victorian Culture*, Harvard University Press, Boston.

HAMILTON, D. (1981) *The Healers: a History of Medicine in Scotland*, Canongate.

HARRISON, M. and ROYSTON, O.M. (1963) *How They Lived, Volume II: an Anthology of Original Accounts written between 1485 and 1700*, Blackwell.

HELLBERG, H. (1983) Health for Some by the year 2000, *People*, **10**, 2, pp. 10–12.

HELLER, R. (1976) 'Priest-Doctors' as a Rural Health Service in the Age of Enlightenment, *Medical History*, **20**, pp. 361–383.

HERZEN, A. (1980 edn) *Childhood, Youth and Exile*, Oxford edn, Oxford University Press.

HMSO (1944) *A National Health Service*, command paper no. 6502, HMSO.

HMSO, (1976) *Fit for the Future — Report of the Committee on Child Health Services (The Court Report)*, Vol. 1, command paper no. 6684, HMSO.

HOBSBAWM, E.J. (1962) *The Age of Revolution, 1789–1848*, Mentor, New York.

HOBSBAWM, E.J. (1968) *Industry and Empire*, Weidenfeld and Nicolson.

HODGKINSON, R. (1967) *The Origins of the National Health Service*, Wellcome Historical Medical Library.

HORN, J. (1969) *Away with all Pests*, Monthly Review Press, New York.

HUNT, A. (1978) *The Elderly at Home*, HMSO.

HYDE, G. (1974) *The Soviet Health Service: a Historical and Comparative Study*, Lawrence and Wishart.

JONES, I.G. (1979) *Health, Wealth and Politics in Victorian Wales*, University College of Swansea.

JONES, K. (1972) *A History of the Mental Health Services*, Routledge and Kegan Paul.

KEYNES, J.M. (1936) *The General Theory of Employment, Interest and Money*, Cambridge University Press.

KLEIN, R. (1983) *The Politics of the National Health Service*, Longman.

LASLETT, P. (1979) *The World We Have Lost*, Methuen.

LAST, J.M. (1963) The Iceberg: 'Completing the Clinical Picture in General Practice', *Lancet*, **2**, pp. 28–31.

LOCKYER, R. (1964) *Tudor and Stuart Britain 1471–1714*, Longman.

LOUDON, I. (1978) Historical Importance of Outpatients, *British Medical Journal*, 15 April, pp. 974–977.

MCDONALD, D. (1950) *Surgeons Twoe and a Barber*, Heinemann.

MACKINTOSH, J.M. (1953) *Trends of Opinion about the Public Health, 1901–1951*, Oxford University Press.

MAGGS, C.J. (1983) *The Origins of General Nursing*, Croom Helm.

MAIR, G.B. (1974) *Confessions of a Surgeon*, William Luscombe.

MARTIN, J. and ROBERTS, C. (1984) *Women and Employment: a Lifetime Perspective*, OPCS/HMSO.

MARX, K. and ENGELS, F. (1965 edn) *The German Ideology*, Lawrence and Wishart.

MAXWELL, R. (1981) *Health and Wealth: An International Study of Health-Care Spending*, D.C. Heath.

MAYNARD, A. and LUDBROOK, A. (1981) Thirty Years of Fruitless Endeavour? An Analysis of Government Intervention in the Health Care Market, in J. Van der Gaag and M. Perlman (eds) *Health, Economics, and Health Economics*, North-Holland, Amsterdam.

MEJIA, A., PIZURKI, H. and ROYSTON, E. (1979) *Physician and Nurse Migration: Analysis and Policy Implications*, WHO, Geneva.

MILLS, A. (1983) Vertical versus Horizontal Health Programs in Africa, *Social Science and Medicine*, **17**, 24, pp. 1971–1981.

MORROW, R.H. (1983) A Primary Health Care Strategy for Ghana, in D. Morley, G.E. Rohde, and G. Williams (eds) *Practising Health for All*, Oxford University Press.

NABARRO, D. (1982) Health for All by the Year 2000: a Great Polemic dissolves into Platitudes? Unpublished lecture delivered at the London School of Hygiene and Tropical Medicine.

NEUGEBAUER, R (1978) Treatment of the Mentally Ill in Medieval and Early Modern England, *Journal of the History of Behavioural Sciences*, **14**, pp. 158–169.

NEWHOUSE, J.P. (1977) Medical Care Expenditure: a cross-national Survey, *Journal of Human Resources*, **12**, 1, pp. 115–125.

NEWMAN, C. (1957) in F.N.L. Poynter (ed.) *The Evolution of Medical Education in Britain*, Pitman Medical.

NISSEL, M. and BONNERJEA, L. (1982) *Family Care of the Handicapped Elderly: Who Pays?*, Paper no. 602, Policy Studies Institute.

OECD (Organization for Economic Co-operation and Development) (1977) *Public Expenditure on Health*, OECD, Paris.

OHE (Office of Health Economics) (1968) *Without Prescription: a Study of the Role of Self-Medication*, OHE.

PASQUINO, P. (1978) Theatricum Politicum. The Genealogy of capital — Police and the State of Prosperity, *Ideology and Consciousness*, **4**, pp. 41–54.

PATTERSON, T. (1983) Science and Medicine in India, in P. Corsi and P. Weindling (eds), *Information Sources in the History of Science and Medicine*, pp. 457–475, Butterworth.

PELLING, M. (1985a) Healing the Sick Poor: Social Policy and Disability in Norwich 1550–1640, *Medical History*, **29**, pp. 115–137

PELLING, M. (1985b) Appearance and Reality: Barbersurgeons, the Body and Disease in early modern London, in L. Beier and R. Finlay (eds) (1985) *The Making of the Metropolis*, Longman.

PELLING, M. and WEBSTER, C. (1979) Medical Practitioners, in C. Webster (ed.) (1979) *Health, Medicine and Mortality in the Sixteenth Century*, pp. 165–235, Cambridge University Press.

PEP (Political and Economic Planning) (1944) Medical Care for Citizens, *Planning*, no. 222.

PHILLIPS, A. and RAKUSEN, J. (eds) (1979) see 'Boston Women's Health Book Collective'.

PHILLIPS, E.D. (1973) *Greek Medicine*, Thames and Hudson.

PIACHAUD, D. (1979) The Diffusion of Medical Techniques to less developed Countries, *International Journal of Health Services*, **9**, 4, pp. 629–643.

POUNDS, N.J.G. (1974) *An Economic History of Medieval Europe*, Longman.

PRINCE, J. (1984) Education for a Profession: some Lessons from History, *International Journal of Nursing Studies*, **21**, 3, pp. 153–163.

RAMALINGASWARMI, P. (1973) India, in I. Douglas-Wilson and G. McLachlan (eds) *Health Service Prospects: An International Survey*, Nuffield Provincial Hospitals Trust.

RAWCLIFFE, C. (1984) The Hospitals of later Medieval London, *Medical History*, **28**, pp. 1–21.

RIFKIN, S. and KAPLINSKY, R. (1973) Health Strategy and Development Planning: Lessons from the People's Republic of China, *Journal of Development Studies*, **9**, 2, pp. 213–232.

ROBERTS, E. (1980) Oral History Investigation of Disease and its Management by the Lancashire Working Class 1890–1939, in J.V. Pickstone (ed.) *Health, Disease and Medicine in Lancashire 1750–1950*, University of Manchester Institute of Technology.

ROEMER, M. and SCHWARTZ, J. (1979) Doctor Slowdown: Effects on the Population of Los Angeles County, *Social Science and Medicine*, **13c**, pp. 213–218.

ROSEN, G. (1958) *A History of Public Health*, MD Publications, New York.

ROSEN, G. (1963) The Hospital: Historical Sociology of a Community Institution, in E. Freidson (ed.) *The Hospital in Modern Society*, pp. 1–36, Free Press, Collier-Macmillan.

ROWLAND, B. (1981) *Medieval Woman's Guide to Health: The First English Gynaecological Handbook* (reproduced and translated from manuscript Sloane 2463) Croom Helm.

RUBIN, S. (1974) *Medieval English Medicine*, Barnes and Noble.

SAI, F. (1973) Ghana, in I. Douglas-Wilson and G. McLachlan (eds) *Health Service Prospects: An International Survey*, Nuffield Provincial Hospitals Trust.

SAVAGE-SMITH, E. (1985). *History of Medieval Islamic Medicine*, Centre Nationale de la Recherche Scientifique, Paris, forthcoming.

SCAMBLER, A., SCAMBLER, G. and CRAIG, D. (1981) Kinship and Friendship and Women's Demand for Primary Care, *Journal of the Royal College of General Practitioners*, **31**, pp. 746–750.

SCULL, A. (1979) *Museums of Madness: The Social Organization of Insanity in Nineteenth-century England*, Allen Lane.

SIGERIST, H. (1943) From Bismarck to Beveridge: Developments and Trends in Social Security Legislation, *Bulletin of the History of Medicine*, **13**, pp. 365–388.

SIMON, J. (1890, reprinted 1970) *English Sanitary Institutions, Reviewed in their Course of Developments, and in some of their Political and Social Relations*, Cassell, reprinted Johnson, New York.

SMITH, A. (1976 edn) *An Inquiry into the Nature and Causes of the Wealth of Nations*, vol. I of the Glasgow edition, R.H. Campbell and A.S. Skinner (eds), Oxford University Press.

SMITH, F.B. (1979) *The People's Health 1830–1910*, Croom Helm.

STARR, P. (1982) *The Social Transformation of American Medicine*, Basic Books, New York.

STOECKLE, J. (1984) The Search for the Healthy Body, *Social Science and Medicine*, **18**, pp. 707–712.

TAYLOR, A.J.P. (1965) *English History 1914–1945*, Oxford University Press.

TIMES ATLAS OF THE WORLD, see Barraclough (1984).

TAYLOR, R. and RIEGER, A. (1984) Rudolf Virchow on the Typhus Epidemic in Upper Silesia: an Introduction and Translation, *Sociology of Health and Illness*, **6**, pp. 201–217.

THOMAS, E.G. (1980) The Old Poor Law and Medicine, *Medical History*, **24**, pp. 1–19.

TITMUSS, R. (1950) *Problems of Social Policy*, HMSO.

TITMUSS, R. (1976) *Essays on the 'Welfare State'* (3rd edn), Allen and Unwin.

TOCQUEVILLE, A. DE (ed. J. Mayer, 1958) *Recollections of A. de Tocqueville*, Meridian.

TURNER, E.S. (1958) *Call the Doctor: A Social History of Medical Men*, Michael Joseph.

UNDERWOOD, E.A. (1977) *Boerhaave's Men at Leyden and After*, Edinburgh University Press.

WADDINGTON, I. (1985) *The Medical Profession in the Industrial Revolution*, Gill and Macmillan.

WATKIN, B. (1975) *Documents on Health and Social Services: 1834 to the Present Day*, Methuen.

WEBSTER, C. (1975) *The Great Instauration*, Duckworth.

WEBSTER, C. (1978) The Crisis of the Hospitals in the Industrial Revolution in E.G. Forbes (ed.) *Human Implications of Scientific Advance*, pp. 214–233, Edinburgh University Press.

WEEKS, J. (1981) *Sex, Politics and Society: the Regulation of Sexuality since 1800*, Longman.

WHITE, L. (1976) The Expansion of Technology 500–1500, in C.M. Cipolla (ed.) *The Middle Ages*, Harvester.

WHO (World Health Organization) (1981) *Health Services in Europe*, vol. 1, WHO, Copenhagen.

WINSLOW, C.E.A. (1920) The Untilled Fields of Public Health, *Modern Medicine*, **2**, pp. 183–191.

WITTS, L.J. (1971) The Medical Professional Unit (The Harveian Oration of 1971), *British Medical Journal*, **4**, pp. 319–323.

WOHL, A. (1983) *Endangered Lives: Public Health in Victorian Britain*, Dent.

WOODHAM-SMITH, C. (1951) *Florence Nightingale*, Penguin.

WOODWARD, J. (1974) *To Do the Sick No Harm: a Study of the British Voluntary Hospital System to 1875*, Routledge and Kegan Paul.

WORLD BANK (1984) *World Development Report, 1984*, Oxford University Press.

WORLDWATCH (1981) Infant Mortality and the Health of Societies, *Worldwatch*, paper no. 47.

WRIGHT, K., CAIRNS, J. and SNELL, M. (1981) *Costing Care*, University of Sheffield.

WYMAN, A.L. (1984) The Surgeoness: the Female Practitioner of Surgery 1400–1800, *Medical History*, **28**, pp. 22–41.

Further reading

BARRACLOUGH, G. (ed.) (1985, 2nd edn) *The Times Atlas of World History*, Times Books.

Lavish maps and concise commentaries covering a very wide range of historical periods, topics and areas of the world. Excellent first port of call for general reference and browsing.

CORSI, P. and WEINDLING, P. (eds) (1983) *Information Sources in the History of Science and Medicine*, Butterworth.

A compendious bibliographical reference book with international coverage and a valuable series of commentaries by subject-area specialists.

DONNELLY, M. (1985) *Managing the Mind: a Study of Medical Psychology in early Nineteenth-Century Britain*, Tavistock.

An interesting modern account of the emergence of psychiatry.

DONNISON, J. (1977) *Midwives and Medical Men*, Schocken Books, New York.

An historical account of inter-personal rivalries and women's rights in one area of health care. Mainly UK oriented.

DOYAL, L. and PENNELL, I. (1979) *The Political Economy of Health*, Pluto.

A readable account from a socialist perspective in which international health and health care problems are viewed as attributable largely to the workings of the capitalist system.

ECKSTEIN, H. (1958) *The English Health Service*, Oxford University Press.

An American political scientist looks at the origins and nature of the NHS with the insight of an outsider.

FOUCAULT, M. (1973) *Madness and Civilisation*, Vintage Books; and (1976) *The Birth of the Clinic*, Tavistock.

Michel Foucault, until his death in 1984, was Professor of the History of Systems of Thought at the Collège de France, Paris. He has been a controversial and unsettling influence on a whole range of disciplines — politics, history, social science and philosophy — and, in his unconventional approach to history, health care has had a central place. Thought provoking.

GLASER, W. (1970) *Social Settings and Medical Organization: a Cross-National Study of the Hospital*, Atherton Press, New York.

Hospitals in sixteen countries in 1961–1962 provide the empirical material for this attempt at a theory of comparative organisational sociology. A bit dated, but ambitious and interesting.

HAMILTON, D. (1981) *The Healers: a History of Medicine in Scotland*, Canongate.

An excellent, well-written example of a one-country history that adopts a broad view of health care.

INGLIS, B. (1965) *A History of Medicine*, Weidenfeld and Nicolson.

A popular history, packed with fascinating illustrations.

NAVARRO, V. (1978) *Class Struggle, the State and Medicine*, Martin Robertson.

A Marxist view of medical care developments in Britain from 1911 to the 1970s.

ROSEN, G. (1974) *From Medical Police to Social Medicine: Essays on the History of Health Care*, Science History Publications, New York.

A fascinating and wide-ranging collection of essays from a leading medical historian.

SMITH, F. B. (1979) *The People's Health, 1830–1910*, Croom Helm.

This book displays all the advantages of a history written from the point of view of ordinary people. A wealth of extraordinary information and an extensive bibliography.

WATKIN, B. (1975) *Documents on Health and Social Services: 1834 to the Present Day*, Methuen.

Watkin collected together in this book extracts from all the important official publications in the UK over the last 150 years, accompanied by a clear and digestible commentary.

Places to visit

The Wellcome Museum of the History of Medicine has the most extensive collection in the world relating to medicine and health care history, including many artefacts, instruments, operating theatres, etc. A permanent display can be seen at the Science Museum, Exhibition Road, London, SW7 2DD. Well worth a visit.

Answers to self-assessment questions

Chapter 2

1 Hippocratic medicine was naturalistic; that is, it considered disease could be explained and understood in terms of natural rather than supernatural events. Whereas Aesculapian medicine relied entirely on suggestion and belief, the Hippocratic school was based on reason and observation. Aesculapians could only effect 'cures' if patients went to the temple, where the ceremony and rituals induced hope and awe. In contrast the Hippocratics travelled from town to town equipped only with their knowledge, books and simple instruments. While they too relied to some extent on suggestion (the placebo effect), Hippocratic medicine represented a fundamental shift by locating disease in the natural rather than the supernatural world.

2 There is no doubt that the Greeks were aware of the importance of environmental factors on the state of health of the population. For example, the Hippocratic work *Airs, Waters and Places* reveals the extent of their knowledge. The main reason usually cited for their failure to translate such knowledge into practical measures, when compared with the Romans, was their lack of systematic social organisation. This, combined with technological developments achieved by the Romans (such as the construction of arches), provided them with the means of accomplishing massive engineering works such as baths and sewers.

3 Christianity favoured the family of God and the Church in place of the 'biological' family of parents and other relatives. In the early medieval period, the spread of Christianity led to the Church accumulating vast wealth, a part of which was used to provide health care and welfare for people. Some of these people may have originally been impoverished by their ancestors giving their wealth to the Church.

4 The newly emerging towns of the eleventh century onwards were far from healthy places to live, but there were in fact repeated attempts to improve the environment. Many sanitary regulations were established, though the extent to which they were observed by the growing urban population is unclear. Whereas the Roman Empire had concentrated on massive constructions, the period from the seventh to the fourteenth centuries achieved little in the way of public engineering. Whether such measures would have made any difference to the epidemics, such as plague, which swept across Europe during that time, is doubtful.

5 The Islamic world played a crucial role in the development of European health care. With the fall of Rome, and later of Christian Constantinople, the European tradition passed into Muslim hands where it was further developed in several ways. The hospital grew into an ever more complex organisation; Greek and Roman knowledge was mixed with that of other traditions, such as Indian. In the late medieval period these developments returned to Europe through the construction of Islamic hospitals, such as those in Spain, and through the new universities, such as the one at Salerno.

Chapter 3

1 The Poor Law Acts were motivated by reasons such as (i) maintaining the strength of the realm; (ii) averting the break-up of villages; and (iii) controlling vagrants and wanderers. Food policies, aimed at ensuring food supplies for the poor, fitted well with all three objectives: (i) averting famine; (ii) overcoming local shortages; and (iii) preventing discontent and wandering destitutes. Taking Poor Law legislation as a parallel, it could be predicted that the effectiveness of such policies would be handicapped by the difficulty of implementing them with the existing administrative apparatus of government, and there is evidence that this indeed was the case.

2 By the 1760s the centre of gravity in British university medical training was decisively in Edinburgh, and large numbers of medical graduates were going to England and elsewhere for employment. In this the London College of Physicians attempted to thwart them by refusing to recognise 'Scotch' degrees. It was this refusal that led to the direct action of storming the college.

3   As the quote from Franklin suggests, one of the factors leading to the development of voluntary hospitals was the increasing awareness of the value to society in financial terms of restoring sick people to health. A second major influence was the medical profession. Medical training, which had been transformed by Boerhaave at Leyden, combined with changes in scientific thinking, led to medicine separating the sick who might be 'restored to health and comfort' from the other inmates of the traditional hospitals. Also, the development of large urban populations meant that large hospitals could be created in which the study of disease and the teaching of medicine could be carried out.

Chapter 4

1   The social and economic conditions of people's lives. Virchow had demonstrated such an association in his report on conditions in Upper Silesia. Similarly, Villermé had studied the relationship between living conditions and mortality in Paris. Both Virchow and Simon believed that significant health improvements could only be brought about by changes in social and economic structures through political intervention. But whereas Virchow was interested in the overthrow of the existing order, Simon was more concerned to expand and modify the existing system of poor relief and public health.

2   There was little state involvement. As you can see in the extract from the directory, only one of the practitioners (J. Breach) was employed by the state, as surgeon to a Poor Law Union. Of the other two, one was an élite surgeon, trained in Europe and working and teaching in a voluntary hospital, while the other was an apothecary, dispensing eggs alongside health care.

In the latter half of the nineteenth century state involvement increased. The 1858 Medical Act established a state licensing system. The development of state involvement in caring for the sick poor, in public health and in providing asylums for the insane all required the employment of doctors.

3   The examples we included, such as the Salford Health Week, the establishment of the Central Council for Health Education, and the campaign to reduce venereal disease, all suggest that health education became more pronounced in the 1920s and 1930s, although you also saw that the health visitors were active long before this period. Public health in the nineteenth century was oriented towards the control and regulation of the environment, but in the early twentieth century, particularly in the aftermath of the Boer War, the state began to pay more attention to issues of personal health. This move would fit with an increasing governmental emphasis on personal health education.

4   You might have mentioned some of the following: the rapid spread of public baths and laundries; the mass manufacture, marketing and advertising of soap; the wider availability of printed books and manuals; and the development of a proprietary medicine industry which may have begun to erode the popularity of traditional medicines and ointments.

5   The 1911 National Health Insurance Scheme closely resembled the German scheme in this respect. And, as later parts of the chapter showed, a large though falling number of societies continued to operate the British scheme right up to the Second World War.

6   (i) The status of the voluntary hospitals generally was much higher, because they included in their numbers the main teaching and specialist hospitals. Poor Law hospitals, even when well-run, were tainted by their association with the workhouse.

(ii) The Poor Law hospitals contained a much larger number of beds than the voluntary hospitals, although in the inter-war period the voluntary system was growing more rapidly.

(iii) Standards of care are more difficult to compare, because the voluntary hospitals tended to concentrate on acute work, whereas the Poor Law hospitals had also to deal with chronic and infectious diseases. The voluntary hospitals certainly had more trained nurses compared with the Poor Law hospitals, and by the 1920s and 1930s many of the voluntary hospitals were probably in better financial shape than Poor Law hospitals, and could therefore afford higher standards. On the other hand, we noted that by international standards, hospital medicine in British voluntary hospitals was falling behind that in Germany or America, and certain parts of the Poor Law system, for example in London, maintained high standards.

Chapter 5

1   The quote illustrates the degree to which all civilians were involved in the war. Health and social policy measures reflected this widening involvement through more comprehensive health services such as the Emergency Medical Service, and it can be inferred that social policy measures also widened (as in fact they did) to cover housing policy, evacuation, relocation and resettlement.

2   Hospital doctors were broadly in favour of the NHS, believing that it would improve working conditions. They were opposed to local authority involvement, however. Their views were represented by the Royal Colleges, particularly the Royal College of Physicians. The General practitioners were divided, and although the majority eventually voted in favour and agreed to work with it, the leadership in the British Medical Association continued its opposition until the NHS began.

3 The NHS inherited an ageing hospital stock that was not evenly distributed in relation to the population, and that contained a particularly high proportion of very old mental illness hospitals. General practitioners were also unevenly distributed, and mainly working in single practices. Changing these patterns became important policy objectives of the NHS.

4 Public and environmental health measures effected great improvement in smoke abatement, and increased the legal responsibilities of employers concerning industrial hazards, sickness, and the provision of information. But the rapid technological change in large sectors of industry has repeatedly run ahead of public and environmental health regulation and control.

Chapter 6

1 (i) As in America, most health care in modern Britain still takes place in the lay sector. In one British study only one woman in sixty consulted a doctor about a headache, only one in eleven about stomach pains. In another study, 88 per cent of those attending a general practitioner had consulted someone else before seeking formal care. Books and magazines too were consulted, though on a smaller scale — 16 per cent of those visiting the GP had tried this. As for self-prescribed drugs, in a study of one British town 15 per cent of adults had taken them in the last two days (a figure that is very similar to the 18 per cent who had done so in a town in the USA).
   (ii) Lay nursing care.

2 Lay care of the dependent is 'cheaper' than institutional care because it relies primarily on the unpaid labour of women. Most lay care is done by women and in a national survey by the Department of Employment in Britain, one in seven women were currently caring for someone such as a sick or elderly relative. The cost of this to the state is kept down because only a small number qualify for the Invalid Care Allowance, and married and cohabiting women are entirely excluded.

3 (i) The 'clinical iceberg' is a phrase that implies there is a vast amount of illness which doctors do not currently see and which they could treat better if only they could get to it. It therefore justifies further intervention into the lay sector by experts. Those who stress the disadvantages of a monopoly of expertise are more likely to appeal to the notion of an 'iceberg' of health care because this image pays explicit attention to the vast amount of lay care that currently receives little official recognition. The notion of a 'clinical iceberg', by contrast, is likely to be unattractive to them, since it implies that while the lay sector may be vast the competence of its workers is limited, and since it implies the furtherance of expert monopoly.

Chapter 7

1 In the seventeenth and eighteenth centuries, many Europeans were fascinated by non-European indigenous health care. Plants and other remedies were studied, collected and brought back to Europe. By the nineteenth century this interest appears to have waned. European health care steadily supplanted indigenous care, at least for the powerful élites. In some countries, such as Thailand and Japan, this transition was remarkably rapid.

2 An increase in the number of doctors being produced in the UK would, in a few years time, mean that there would be less demand for doctors to come to the UK from India and other countries. If this meant that there were then too many doctors in India, some could find themselves unemployed unless some other recipient country was available.

Chapter 8

1 Health insurance has historical roots in societies and funds that were often begun by specific occupational groups, or religious bodies, etc. These were discussed in Chapter 4. There you also saw that in Germany after 1883 and Britain after 1911 it proved easier to let these many separate organisations continue, even within a national health insurance framework.

2 No. The evidence from international comparisons suggests that as national wealth increases, the *proportion* of it spent on formal health care increases. In other words, each 1 per cent increase in national wealth tends on average to result in more than a 1 per cent increase in formal health care spending.

3 Where fee-for-service payment operates, as you saw, researchers have suggested the existence of a phenomenon known as supplier-induced demand: because the supplier (e.g. a doctor) has more information at her or his disposal, she or he can in effect decide how much of their own services to 'demand'. If financial incentives exist to increase the amount of care supplied, the phenomenon is reinforced. Thus attempts to overcome a 'shortage' of doctors by increasing their number could result in even more demand being generated for their services, and the 'shortage' continuing.

4 First, it is difficult to measure accurately the amount of formal health care in one country compared with another. Second, mortality rates are a measure of death, not health, and it may be that many formal health care activities improve health — by treating disability or easing pain or discomfort — without reducing mortality rates. Third, as previous chapters in the book have also pointed out, there may be many reasons for altering the amount of formal health care that have little to do with either health or

mortality, for example, as an electoral tactic. And fourth, a good deal of health care may operate at the 'margins of the impossible'.

Chapter 9

1   The Dawson report envisaged health centres at a *primary* level, *secondary* health centres providing general in-patient care, and specialised or *tertiary* regional teaching hospitals. So it was an important early example of planning based on this model, the only anomaly being that the primary health centres had in-patient facilities.

2   The first was that vertical programmes often were made untenable by depending on foreign aid, technology and support. The second was that a lack of local involvement in such programmes meant that people could not continue to implement vertical programme activities in the often lengthy spells between visits by centrally-directed programme workers; they were made dependent upon visiting workers.

Index

Acknowledgements

Grateful acknowledgement is made to the following sources for material used in this book.

Text

P. S. Byrne and B. E. L. Lang, *Doctors Talking to Patients*, 1976, reproduced by permission of the Controller of HMSO.

Tables

Table 3.1 C. M. Cipolla, *Public Health and the Medical Profession in the Renaissance*, Cambridge University Press, 1976.

Figures

Figures 1.1 (a and b), 2.3 (a and b), 2.4, 2.11, 3.2, 3.5, 3.7, 4.1, 4.4, 4.7, 4.11 and 6.3 Wellcome Institute Library; *Figures 2.1, 2.10, 2.12, 3.4, 3.6, 4.5, 4.9, 4.13, 5.1 and 7.2* BBC Hulton Picture Library; *Figure 2.5* Museum of Antiquities of Newcastle University and the Society of Antiquaries of Newcastle-upon-Tyne; *Figure 2.6* courtesy of Deutches Museum, Munich; *Figure 2.7* British Museum; *Figure 2.8* courtesy of the Master of Lord Leycester Hospital; *Figure 2.9* British Library; *Figure 4.3* National Portrait Gallery; *Figure 4.4* C. Webster, *The Great Instauration*, Duckworth, 1975; *Figure 4.10 Illustrated London News*; *Figure 4.12* Durham Miners Association; *Figure 5.3* courtesy of *Punch*, 3 April 1946; *Figure 5.5* Keystone; *Figure 7.1* Mansell; *Figure 7.3 Illustrated London News*; *Figure 7.4* Richard Davies; *Figures 8.1 and 9.4* Camerapix Hutchison Library; *Figures 9.1 and 9.2* Novosti; *Figure 9.3 A Primary Health Care Strategy*, Ministry of Health, Ghana, 1978; *Figure 9.5* WHO, *Primary Health Care: The Universal Experience*, WHO, 1983; *Figure 9.6* Monica Boggust of the BBC.

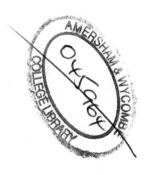